Growing Fruit Trees

Comprehensive Steps for a Healthy Harvest

(A Comprehensive Guide to Starting Fruit Trees From Seed at Home)

John Burton

Published By **Cathy Nedrow**

John Burton

All Rights Reserved

Growing Fruit Trees: Comprehensive Steps for a Healthy Harvest (A Comprehensive Guide to Starting Fruit Trees From Seed at Home)

ISBN 978-1-9994256-6-1

Legal & Disclaimer

Table Of Contents

Chapter 1: Fruit Gardening

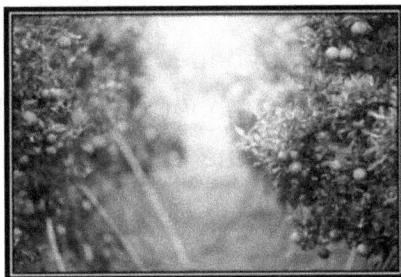

Have you ever dreamed of developing your personal fruit timber? It's now not as tough as you may likely expect. In a global in which immediate gratification and comfort have turn out to be the norm, there may be something deeply profitable approximately tending to the surrender stop result of your tough paintings. Imagine entering into your out of doors and being greeted thru the colorful shades of luscious end result putting from wood, timber, and vines you have got were given carefully nurtured.

Growing quit stop end result can convey you good sized pleasure and fruitful effects. The presence of fruit timber no longer handiest blesses you with a regular deliver of smooth and extremely good produce however furthermore brings about countless blessings to your well-being, the environment, and the humans round you.

Health Benefits

Enhanced Nutritional Value: When you develop your private fruit, you are making sure that each piece you harvest is full of important vitamins, minerals, and antioxidants. Homegrown fruits are identified to be greater nutrient-rich than commercially produced ones, as you have manipulate over cultivation strategies and can select herbal practices and herbal fertilizers. This technique you and your own family can enjoy fruits bursting with goodness, promoting better regular fitness and well-being.

Boosted Immunity: The abundance of vitamins in homegrown surrender end end result contributes to a reinforced immune tool. Vitamin C, located in higher portions in herbal end result, lets in fend off infections and permits a healthy immune response. By eating those fruits frequently, you could enhance your frame's capability to combat off illnesses and live resilient.

Improved Digestion: Homegrown cease result are fresher and masses less possibly to have handed via chemical treatments, making them a whole lot less difficult on your digestive device. The fiber content fabric in those give up give up result aids in better digestion, assisting prevent issues like constipation and selling a greater in shape gut.

Natural Detoxification: The antioxidants observed in homegrown give up quit end result play a critical feature in detoxifying your body. These powerful compounds assist neutralize risky free radicals, decreasing oxidative pressure and helping the body's herbal cleansing tactics.

Mental Well-being: Nurturing a fruit lawn can also have superb outcomes to your highbrow fitness. Spending time outdoor, tending to flowers, and witnessing the fruits of your hard paintings can reduce stress and tension stages. The sense of success you sense while harvesting your homegrown fruits brings a experience of pride and success, fostering a more effective mind-set.

Enhanced Hydration: Freshly harvested end end result are filled with water, imparting a scrumptious and herbal way to stay hydrated. Staying properly-hydrated is crucial for maximum green physical skills, pores and pores and skin health, and keeping strength levels inside the path of the day.

Environmental Sustainability

Biodiversity Preservation: Creating a fruit lawn contributes to biodiversity, attracting numerous pollinators which includes bees and butterflies. These pollinators play a crucial feature in supporting the surroundings, assisting inside the replica of plants, and

4

promoting the survival of neighborhood flora and fauna.

Reduced Carbon Footprint: By developing your fruit, you decrease the selection for for commercially produced give up result requiring large transportation. This reduction in transportation results in a lower carbon footprint, supporting fight climate exchange and shield the surroundings.

Sustainable Gardening Practices: Embracing sustainable gardening practices, which includes composting, rainwater harvesting, and using herbal fertilizers, reduces your garden's impact on the environment. These practices sell more healthful soil, hold water, and reduce the usage of unstable chemicals.

Self-Sufficiency

Food Security: Growing your very own fruit empowers you to take manipulate of your food supply, contributing on your circle of relatives's food protection. You now not totally depend upon external property on your fruit goals, ensuring which you have fresh, homegrown produce absolutely available.

Cost Savings: Cultivating your fruit garden can bring about terrific fee financial savings ultimately. The investment in seeds or younger flowers and soil training is minimum as compared to the continuing fees of buying stop result from shops. Homegrown stop result additionally provide a very precise opportunity to strive uncommon or uniqueness kinds without breaking the monetary organization.

Connection with Nature: Being a solo mother does no longer mean you cannot have a deep reference to nature. Growing your non-public fruit fosters a experience of closeness with the environment. Spending time outdoors, nurturing your plant life, and witnessing the increase of your fruit timber nurtures a greater appreciation for the herbal international.

Skill Development: Taking care of your fruit lawn offers an opportunity to look at and broaden new capabilities in horticulture and gardening. This arms-on experience can be enjoyable and empowering, imparting you with a treasured capability set for self-sufficiency and resilience.

This e-book is a whole manual a great way to take you on a adventure of exploration, empowering you to broaden your very personal fruit and gain a multitude of rewards. By delving into the pages earlier, you may liberate a treasure trove of information and realistic advice to help you domesticate a bountiful fruit garden.

Within those chapters, you could discover the myriad advantages of growing your very non-public fruit. First and most important, you'll find out about the widespread health advantages that sit up for you. Fresh, homegrown fruit gives unparalleled taste, bursting with flavors and textures that surpass what you locate in stores. As you're taking satisfaction in each chew, you could take solace in know-how which you are nourishing your body with nutrient-wealthy produce, harvested at the peak of ripeness for optimum dietary price.

Beyond personal health, you may moreover delve into the environmental sustainability issue of fruit gardening. By tending in your non-public fruit lawn, you're making a contribution to reducing CO_2 emissions through manner of getting rid of or minimizing the need for transportation. This sustainable desire moreover promotes biodiversity as your lawn becomes a haven for pollinators and distinctive useful creatures, fostering a more match ecosystem.

To manual you on this fruitful adventure, this ebook is thoughtfully prepared into severa sections. You will embark on an exploration of fruit cultivation, wherein you can benefit a deep information of plant anatomy and body shape because it relates to fruit production. You may be added to diverse styles of fruit wooden and flora, empowering you to make informed alternatives at the same time as selecting kinds to your lawn.

The significance of careful making plans and format isn't unnoticed. You will find out methods to analyze the to be had place and assets in your fruit lawn, and expertly format a layout that maximizes performance and aesthetic enchantment. Equipped with a seasonal plan for planting and harvesting, you'll make sure a non-prevent supply of scrumptious end result in some unspecified time in the future of the twelve months.

Nurturing the inspiration of your fruit lawn, the e-book delves into soil guidance and nutrient management. You will discover ways to examine soil awesome, beautify fertility, and shape to create an most suitable growing surroundings for your fruit timber and plants. Understanding the dietary goals of your loved one garden population will ensure their robust increase and sufficient fruit manufacturing.

A critical detail of fruit gardening is propagation. You will find out diverse strategies, such as seed propagation, grafting, and budding strategies. Armed with this information, you can with a bit of success propagate your very very own fruit flowers, choosing the suitable approach for every variety and following step-thru using-step instructions for a achievement propagation.

With the foundation laid, you could project into the place of planting and organising fruit wooden. Discover the secrets and techniques and strategies and techniques to choosing wholesome nursery inventory, planting within the right season, and fostering right root improvement. As your timber grow, you can research the artwork of pruning and training, expertise the significance of shaping wood for most efficient productiveness and common tree health.

Maintaining the well-being of your fruit lawn is vital for prolonged-time period achievement. You will delve into vital subjects which include watering and irrigation strategies, pest and illness manipulate using herbal methods, and right fertilization practices. Armed with this knowledge, you can nurture your lawn with care, making sure thriving fruit timber and delicious yields.

As the end end result of your exertions begin to ripen, you may observe the artwork of harvesting and keeping. Discover the best strategies for figuring out fruit ripeness and dealing with harvested fruit to maintain tremendous and freshness. Explore pretty a variety of protection techniques, from canning and freezing to dehydrating and making preserves, allowing you to have a laugh with the flavors of your lawn 365 days-round.

This e-book goes beyond the ordinary, exploring distinctiveness give up give up end result and uncommon types. From figs to pomegranates and persimmons, you may release the secrets and techniques and techniques of cultivating the ones specific treasures, growing your fruit garden collection, and tantalizing your taste buds with their brilliant flavors.

With expertise comes the functionality to triumph over demanding conditions. You can be equipped with precious insights into identifying and dealing with common pests, illnesses, and troubles that may rise up in your fruit garden. Troubleshooting nutrient deficiencies, imbalances, and addressing environmental factors will make sure your fruit garden flourishes below any scenario.

As a fruit gardener, your ardour is aware of no obstacles. This e-book embraces the variety of climates and environments, offering hints and techniques for adapting fruit cultivation practices to precise areas. Whether you're residing in a cold or heat climate, metropolis setting, or restrained area, you'll learn how to tailor your fruit garden for your specific conditions.

The paintings of espalier, with its severa benefits, awaits your exploration. Uncover the idea of espalier and take a look at step-with the aid of-step commands for education fruit wooden in lovely espalier paperwork. From conventional designs to revolutionary variations, espalier techniques will add a hint of beauty and area-saving capability to your fruit lawn.

As your fruit timber mature, you may acquire the skills critical for his or her renewal and prolonged-time period safety. Techniques for rejuvenating older or left out fruit trees, pruning and shaping mature wooden for endured productiveness, and techniques for ongoing care will make sure the sustainability and abundance of the one that you love fruit garden.

Finally, this ebook ventures into the destiny, exploring sustainable practices and enhancements in fruit gardening. You will discover the location of natural gardening standards, lowering chemical inputs and embracing environmentally pleasant strategies. Explore permaculture, biodynamics, and agroforestry, and witness the capacity they keep for remodeling your fruit garden proper right into a sustainable paradise.

Exploring the Joy and Satisfaction of Cultivating Your Own Fruit

Exploring the joy and delight of cultivating your very very own fruit is a adventure that transcends the mere act of gardening. It is an experience that fills your coronary coronary heart with a feel of accomplishment and fulfillment. As you cautiously nurture your fruit vegetation from tiny seeds or saplings to robust bushes bearing luscious end give up result, you emerge as in element linked with the natural global.

There is a profound sense of pleasure that comes from witnessing the increase and transformation of your fruit lawn. From the primary smooth buds to the colourful blossoms that supply in the appearance of fruit, every diploma of the way brings anticipation and pleasure. The sheer wonder of nature's cycles unfolding in advance than your eyes is genuinely awe-inspiring.

The delight derived from cultivating your personal fruit extends past the mere act of harvest. When you pluck a ripe, juicy fruit from a tree you planted and cared for, a profound experience of gratification washes over you. You become in element privy to the try, time, and self-discipline invested in nurturing that fruit to its top of perfection. Each bite becomes a party of your tough artwork and willpower.

There is a deep-rooted connection amongst people and the act of developing meals. Cultivating your very very own fruit taps into this primal intuition, presenting a tangible link to our ancestors who trusted their very personal arms to hold themselves. In current-day day rapid-paced and disconnected worldwide, tending to a fruit garden brings us lower again to our roots, reminding us of the innate human capability to nurture and offer for ourselves.

Beyond the physical rewards, the joy of cultivating your personal fruit lies in the intangible blessings it brings in your lifestyles. Spending time to your fruit lawn may be a recuperation and rejuvenating enjoy. The sight of vibrant foliage, the fragrance of blossoms, and the moderate breeze rustling thru the branches create a tranquil sanctuary in which you could escape the stresses of every day existence.

Furthermore, cultivating your very own fruit gives a experience of empowerment and self-sufficiency. It allows you to break loose from the dependency on closely produced, keep-bought fruit and take manage of your very very own food deliver. You become an energetic participant in the journey from farm to table, understanding precisely how your fruit come to be grown and the care it acquired.

Chapter 2: Understanding Fruit Cultivation

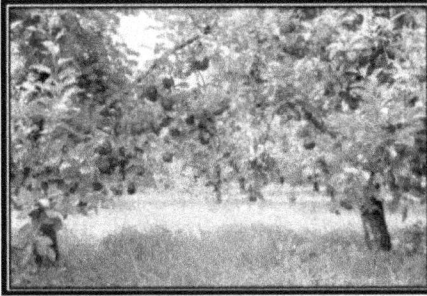

Fruit gardening includes cultivating fruit plants, collectively with the seed-bearing systems observed in flowering flowers and nuts, for business and consumption functions. Surprisingly, simplest one out of every 3 people who expand vegetables furthermore engage in fruit cultivation.

There is a not unusual assumption that fruit gardening is more complicated than vegetable gardening or calls for excessive vicinity, but this isn't actual. Unlike veggies, which need to be planted anew every year, fruit vegetation in truth require ordinary feeding and pruning to maintain productiveness over numerous years.

Basics of Plant Anatomy and Physiology Related to Fruit Production.

Fruits can be categorized into three number one anatomical training, mainly mixture stop cease result, multiple quit result, and easy give up end result. These lessons are primarily based on the mature ovary or ovaries of 1 or greater vegetation. In advantageous fruits, the in form to be eaten issue does now not originate from the ovary itself but as an alternative from the aril. Examples of such fruits include the mangosteen and pomegranate, in which tissues from the flower and stem offer the meals supply, in addition to the pineapple.

When it comes to grasses, their grains are considered unmarried-seed easy give up result. In this form of fruit, the pericarp and seed coat are fused right into a unmarried layer, it definitely is known as a caryopsis. Cereal grains like wheat, barley, oats, and rice are commonplace examples of caryopsis quit end result.

Categories of Fruits

Fruits may be labeled into three crucial anatomical groups: mixture fruits, a couple of give up end result, and easy give up quit result. Aggregate cease cease end result are formed from a single compound flower and include more than one ovaries or fruitlets, along aspect raspberries and blackberries. Multiple cease quit result are created via the usage of the fusion of ovaries from more than one plants or inflorescences, as visible in figs, mulberries, and pineapples. Simple fruits, as an alternative, growth from a unmarried ovary and may incorporate one or severa seeds. They may be every fleshy or dry.

In fleshy fruits, the pericarp and one among a kind accessory systems emerge as the fleshy a part of the fruit at some point of development. Berries, pomes, and drupes are examples of fleshy stop result. Berries have a fleshy pericarp, aside from the exocarp, which acts greater like skin. Some berries, like pepo (e.G., cucumber) or hesperidium (e.G., lemon), have either inseparable or separable rinds. Pomes have a fleshy factor advanced from the floral tube, with most of the pericarp being fleshy but the endocarp being cartilaginous (e.G., apple).

Drupes are one-seeded end result with a fleshy mesocarp (e.G., peach). However, a few stop give up end result, like strawberries, have a fleshy element superior from tissues apart from the ovary. In the case of strawberries, the correct for ingesting component is original from the receptacle of the flower. Such culmination are referred to as faux end result or accessory end result.

Fleshy end result rent a shared method of seed dispersal, relying on animals to eat the fruits and scatter the seeds, therefore making sure the survival of their populations. Dry cease result, but, growth from the ovary but do now not depend upon the mesocarp for seed dispersal. Instead, they depend upon physical forces inclusive of wind and water.

Some dry end result rent pod shattering, in which the seed is forcibly ejected from the seed coat. Others can carry out seed pod explosions, like wisteria, which disperses seeds over extended distances. Similar to fleshy fruits, dry fruits also can rely on animals for seed dispersal via adhering to their fur or pores and skin, a technique called epizoochory.

Dry end result may be further categorized into different types, together with achenes, drugs, follicles, or nuts. They additionally can be labeled as dehiscent or indehiscent fruits. Dry dehiscent culmination have pods that boom inner anxiety, allowing seeds to be launched. Examples of dry dehiscent quit result include sweet peas, soybeans, alfalfa, milkweed, mustard, cabbage, and poppy.

Dry indehiscent end quit result, on the other hand, do no longer non-public this mechanism and rely absolutely on physical forces for dispersal. Species like sunflower seeds, nuts, and dandelions are examples of dry indehiscent culmination.

Pericarp Layer

When it comes to fleshy fruits, the pericarp includes three wonderful layers: the outermost layer referred to as the epicarp or exocarp, the middle layer referred to as the mesocarp, and the inner layer surrounding the ovary or seeds referred to as the endocarp. In citrus culmination, the epicarp and mesocarp together shape the peel. However, in dry fruits, the pericarp layers aren't really distinguishable.

Epicarp:

The epicarp, additionally known as the exocarp or flavedo in citrus culmination, is the outermost layer of the pericarp. It forms the tough outer pores and pores and pores and skin of the fruit, if present.

Mesocarp:

The mesocarp is the fleshy middle layer of the pericarp, decided among the epicarp and the endocarp. It is frequently the a part of the fruit that is consumed. For example, in a peach, the mesocarp makes up the bulk of the in shape to be eaten element, and in a tomato, it contributes drastically to its form. The time period "mesocarp" also can communicate to any fruit this is fleshy in some unspecified time in the future of.

In citrus surrender end result, especially hesperidium culmination, the mesocarp is also known as albedo or pith. It constitutes the internal part of the peel and is commonly eliminated in advance than intake. In citron fruit, wherein the mesocarp is the most high-quality part, it is used within the manufacturing of succade.

Endocarp:

The endocarp is the inner layer of the pericarp that proper away surrounds the seeds. In a few cease end result, such as citrus, it could be membranous and is the handiest thing that is fed on. In one-of-a-kind surrender result like peaches, cherries, plums, and apricots, the endocarp is thick and tough, forming the stony layer known as the pyrenes.

In the case of nuts, the endocarp refers to the difficult layer that surrounds the kernel of pecans, walnuts, and specific comparable nuts, and it is also removed earlier than intake.

In citrus quit end end result, the endocarp is split into segments, frequently referred to as sections, which may be complete of juice vesicles containing the fruit's juice.

Fruit wood embody a extensive sort of flowering timber that yield fruit. When considering the one of a kind sorts of fruit bushes, our minds normally gravitate in the direction of timber that undergo delicious, ripe, sweet, or tangy juicy end result. Apple bushes, pear timber, cherry trees, and plum timber are the various maximum typically located fruit timber in gardens. In regions with warmer climates, fruit-bearing flowers also encompass apricots, peaches, and figs.

From a botanical mind-set, the elegance of fruit trees can encompass wood that produce berries or nuts as well. This is due to the fact stop give up result are scientifically labeled due to the fact the matured ovaries of vegetation that include at the least one seed. Therefore, consistent with botanical terminology, tomatoes, eggplants, peas, and beans are all outstanding styles of cease give up result considering that they're seed-bearing structures.

Chapter 3: Planning Your Fruit Garden

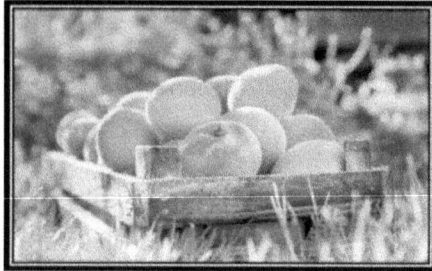

When it includes fruit gardening, you need to anticipate ahead greater than you'll for a vegetable lawn. Fruit-bearing plants, in conjunction with timber or shrubs, have longer lifespan, starting from 10 to 50 years or perhaps extra. Investing some effort and time in making plans and getting prepared your fruit garden is appreciably beneficial as it consequences in large harvests every 12 months with minimal effort and time required.

Assessing the Available Space and Resources for Your Fruit Garden

Evaluate the Location

To begin, thoroughly study the region in which you would like to installation your fruit lawn. Take observe of the daylight exposure, soil type, drainage, and any functionality elements that might impact the increase of your fruit plant life. Pay interest to nearby timber or systems that could strong shade and avoid daylight hours penetration or have an effect on root development.

Measure the Available Space

Accurately measuring the dimensions of your distinct fruit garden vicinity is essential for powerful making plans. By figuring out the size of the space, you may evaluate what number of fruit timber or vegetation you may accommodate and design the ideal format. This step guarantees that your lawn does not turn out to be overcrowded or avoid the wholesome increase of your plants.

Determine Sunlight Requirements

Different fruit wooden and flora have specific daylight requirements. Observe the quantity of daylight your chosen location gets at a few stage inside the day. Ideally, fruit bushes want at the least 6-eight hours of direct daylight each day for pinnacle-rated boom and fruit production. Assess whether or not the vicinity meets those necessities based totally on its publicity to daytime.

Assess Soil Quality

Understanding the composition and satisfactory of your soil is essential for the achievement of your fruit lawn. Fruit flora generally thrive in properly-draining soil with ok fertility. Conduct a soil test to evaluate its pH degree and nutrient content. If the soil exceptional is negative, you can want to improve it with the useful resource of way of incorporating natural rely or the use of raised beds or bins to create an crucial developing environment on your fruit vegetation.

Consider Water Accessibility

Evaluate the proximity of a water deliver for your fruit lawn region. Fruiting plants often require constant and enough watering, in particular in some unspecified time in the future of dry durations, to guide wholesome increase and fruit development. Ensure that a water deliver is resultseasily available for irrigation features, both through a close-by tap, rainwater harvesting machine, or a well-designed watering device.

Check for Potential Obstacles

Identify any potential limitations that would hinder the increase and improvement of your fruit garden. This includes massive timber that cast immoderate shade on the region, nearby structures that preclude daylight hours, or underground utilities that could restriction root boom. Removing or addressing those boundaries earlier will help create an greatest growing environment for your fruit plant life.

Determine the Number of Plants

Based at the available area and daylight hours conditions, cautiously determine on the extensive sort of fruit timber or plant life you can accommodate. Consider the spacing requirements of each fruit range, making sure that there can be incredible enough room for growth and right air go with the flow. Overcrowding can cause opposition for assets and prolonged susceptibility to ailments or pests.

Research Fruit Varieties

Thoroughly studies precise fruit sorts appropriate for your particular climate and developing situations. Take into interest factors including the sort of loosen up hours required for fruit set, pollination requirements (together with pass-pollination if important), sickness resistance, and the ultimate size of mature timber. Choose fruit sorts that align collectively with your options, to be had sources, and the climatic suitability of your region.

Assess Additional Resources

Consider more property that can be important in your fruit garden. These may also moreover moreover embody trellises or stakes for assisting hiking flora, netting for protecting quit result from birds, or fertilizers to beautify soil fertility. Assess whether you already possess those property or in case you want to gather them in advance than starting up your fruit gardening project.

Plan the Layout

Once you have got collected all of the critical data and assessed available belongings, plan the layout of your fruit lawn. Consider the mature period of the plants and allow ok spacing amongst them to make certain advanced increase and improvement. Pay attention to the proximity of properly matched flowers for pass-pollination and plan for ease of protection and harvesting. A nicely-concept-out format promotes wholesome plant increase and allows green care all through the developing season.

Designing an Efficient and Aesthetically Pleasing Layout

Understanding the fruit garden format format is critical earlier than embarking on a fruit gardening journey. The method of designing a fruit garden format can bring delight and pride. With cautious schooling and hobby of the flowers' requirements, it's miles possible to installation a vicinity that is visually appealing and in particular fruitful.

Consider every aesthetics and function at the identical time as deciding on vegetation to your fruit lawn. For instance, you may opt for dwarf varieties of end end result like apples and pears to create appealing borders, on the identical time as taller alternatives like peaches or plums can characteristic privateness presentations. Apart from selecting flora that healthy the to be had area, ensure they are nicely-applicable to your weather and soil situations.

Once you have an idea of the flowers you want, it's time to sketch a lawn layout. Take beneath attention the mature duration of every plant, similarly to their daylight and water necessities. Also, thing in any unique goals, in conjunction with help structures for mountaineering vines or trellises for grapevines, even as planning your format.

Things to Know Before Designing Your Fruit Garden Layout

1.   Plan for one in each of a type types of fruit.

When designing your fruit lawn format, it's vital to maintain in thoughts the space requirements of severa sorts of fruit bushes and flora. Each fruit range has its very own growth behavior and spatial wishes. Some fruit wooden, like apple or pear timber, can grow to be pretty large and require enough vicinity for his or her branches to spread. On the possibility hand, berry wooden or dwarf fruit trees can be greater compact and in shape properly in smaller regions or boxes.

Research the mature period of the fruit kinds you endorse to grow and allocate appropriate sufficient place because of this. Consider elements which includes the peak, unfold, and root tool of every plant. Providing enough room for correct air circulate amongst flowers will assist save you illnesses and sell wholesome boom. Additionally, planning for the future increase of your fruit trees guarantees they have enough region to gain their entire capability and bear ample culmination.

2.   Choose a sunny spot.

Selecting the proper area for your fruit garden is critical, and one of the maximum vital factors to endure in mind is daylight. Fruit timber and flora thrive in sunny spots that get preserve of at least six to eight hours of direct daylight each day. Adequate daylight is crucial for photosynthesis, the technique by way of using which flowers convert daylight into power to provide give up result. Without enough daylight hours, fruit flowers may additionally additionally furthermore warfare to boom and undergo fruit.

When choosing a sunny spot, bear in thoughts factors at the facet of the orientation of your garden, nearby structures or bushes that may solid shadows, and the course of the solar at some level within the day. Observe your out of doors and apprehend the regions with the most daylight hours publicity. These areas can be first-class for planting fruit timber and sun-loving flora like berries, citrus wooden, and stone culmination.

3.   Make positive there is right drainage.

Proper drainage is essential for the fitness of your fruit garden. Poor drainage can reason waterlogged soil, which can suffocate plant roots, sell root rot, and prevent the growth of fruit trees and vegetation. It is important to evaluate the drainage tendencies of your garden area in advance than planting.

To ensure pinnacle drainage, avoid low-mendacity regions where water has a bent to gather or areas with compacted soil that forestalls water from permeating. If your soil has terrible drainage, you can decorate it via the use of incorporating herbal don't forget together with compost or well-rotted manure to decorate its form and water-maintaining ability. Alternatively, raised beds or container gardening can be carried out to create higher drainage conditions.

4. Consider trellises or exclusive facilitates.

Some fruit vegetation, especially vine-like flora together with grapes, tomatoes, or positive varieties of berries, advantage from help systems like trellises, stakes, or cages. These facilitates now not fine help the flora increase upright however also make harvesting much less complicated and maximize location utilization for your garden.

Chapter 4: Soil Preparation And Nutrient Management

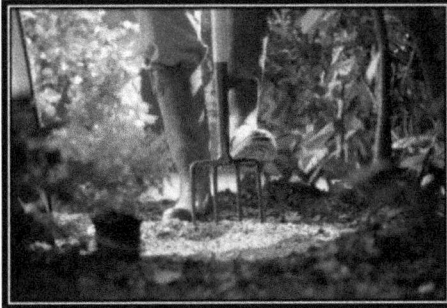

Soil is frequently overlooked and underestimated in its importance. When we encounter a flower we want to plant, we often sincerely dig a hollow, location the flower in it, and assume it to flourish. However, this approach can also simplest be successful with terrific soil great, while the majority people need to alter our soil to installation the proper conditions for gold modern day growth.

Evaluating Soil Quality and Conducting Necessary Soil Tests

Ensuring that your soil has the capability to deliver nutrients to plant life is essential. Otherwise, the increase of your flora could be hindered. Optimal soil pH, which determines acidity stages, is essential for vegetation to take in the required nutrients. If the pH degree is excessively immoderate, vitamins like phosphorus and iron also can grow to be an awful lot lots less handy, even as excessively low pH may be destructive to vegetation. The absence of fertile soil poses a great mission to engaging in a flourishing garden.

Another purpose of soil sorting out is to lessen excessive reliance on fertilizers. By starting off with nutrient-rich soil, the want for giant soil amendments decreases. Prior to using lime and fertilizers, it's far clearly useful to obtain a soil sample for entire analysis.

Conducting a soil take a look at is vital to evaluate the essential tendencies of your soil, which includes its texture (sand, silt, or clay) and acidity diploma (pH). This check additionally determines the supply of essential vitamins like magnesium, calcium, phosphorus, and potassium. Based at the effects, recommendations are provided to adjust every nutrient to the right ranges for most beneficial plant boom. It's crucial to recall that immoderate portions of nutrients may be as harmful as inadequate ranges, so rely upon your soil check as a guide.

For top-satisfactory plant boom, it's far advocated to test your soil's pH and nutrient recognition every three to 5 years. Soil sampling can be completed at any time, but fall is remaining as it allows you to gather consequences and make important changes in advance than spring. While domestic check kits are to be had at gardening centers, they may no longer be as accurate or complete as professional sorting out accomplished through your community county extension administrative center. The correct records is that county extension soil assessments are often unfastened or low-price.

To Obtain a Representative Soil Sample...

Clear the surface of any debris, plant residues, or leaves.

Avoid sampling areas wherein ashes, manure, compost, or brush had been deposited or burned.

Using a shovel or trowel, reduce a V-shaped hole into the soil, approximately 6 to 8 inches deep.

Take a 1-inch massive slice of soil alongside the duration of the hole, and from the center of this slice, acquire a 1-inch strip as your sample.

Repeat this sampling technique randomly throughout your garden, combining the samples in a easy glass jar or bucket. If you have raised beds, take a slice from every mattress and mix them collectively.

Measure out a cupful of soil, permit it dry indoors for a few days, and seal it in a plastic bag categorized along with your data.

Submit the sample with the required paperwork and fees, and appearance in advance on your consequences.

DIY Soil Tests

To gain similarly belief into your soil and its fitness, you can behavior 3 DIY soil checks: assessing soil texture, soil pH, and soil fitness.

1.   Soil Health: The Earthworm Test

The fantastic time to test for earthworms is at a few level within the spring even as the soil temperature reaches 50°F, and the surface is moist. Here's a manner to conduct the test:

Use a shovel to dig up about 1 cubic foot of soil.

Place the soil on a piece of cardboard, destroy it apart, and look for earthworms.

Healthy soil want to have now not less than 10 earthworms. If the variety is decrease, incorporating more herbal count range—on the side of compost, elderly manure, or leaf mildew—is suggested. Organic depend improves soil form, slowly releases vitamins, and complements beneficial microbial activity.

2.   Soil Acidity or Alkalinity: The Pantry Soil pH Test

This test permits you to assess whether or not or not or not your soil is acidic or alkaline:

Place 2 tablespoons of soil in a bowl and upload ½ cup of vinegar. If the mixture fizzes, it indicates alkaline soil.

Place 2 tablespoons of soil in a separate bowl and moisten it with distilled water. Add ½ cup of baking soda. If the combination fizzes, it shows acidic soil.

If there may be no reaction in each test, the soil has a impartial pH.

Extremely immoderate or low pH stages can bring about nutrient deficiency or toxicity in plant life. A pH charge of seven is independent, whilst the form of 5.Five to 7 helps advanced microbial interest and nutrient absorption thru plant roots. Depending on the effects, you can modify the soil pH because of this. Applying finely ground limestone counteracts acidic (sour) soil, at the equal time as ground sulfur treats alkaline (sweet) soil.

3.   Soil Texture: The Peanut Butter Jar Test

This test lets in determine the composition of your soil. Ideally, healthful soil consists of 20% clay, 40% silt, and forty% sand. Follow the ones steps:

Find a right now-sided jar, which encompass a peanut butter or mason jar, with a lid.

Dig all the manner right down to a depth of about 6 inches inside the region you need to check and accumulate sufficient soil to fill the jar to about one-zero.33 or one-1/2.

Fill the jar to the shoulder with water and permit the soil to soak up the water.

Secure the lid tightly and shake the jar vigorously for spherical 3 minutes.

Set the jar apart and, after 1 minute, diploma the sediment settled at the bottom. This shows the sand content material on your soil.

Wait for a similarly four mins and degree the sediment over again. The distinction a few of the measurements suggests the silt content material fabric.

Take a 3rd dimension after 24 hours. The difference the diverse 2nd one and 1/3 measurements represents the clay content material material.

Calculate the possibilities of sand, silt, and clay, which need to normal a hundred%. Loamy soil normally consists of 20% clay, 40% silt, and 40% sand. This test allows you decide which flowers are appropriate for your soil kind. For example, sandy soil drains properly, on the identical time as silt and clay maintain greater moisture, making them ideal for plant life that select wet situations. Accordingly, pick your vegetation or amend the soil therefore.

Techniques for Improving Soil Fertility and Structure

How to Boost Nitrogen Levels

Animal Manure: Different animal species, feed, bedding, and manure storage practices have an impact at the nutrient content cloth material of manure. The availability of nutrients to plants is primarily based upon on the timing and incorporation of manure into the soil. Soil situations furthermore impact nutrient release. Cow manure generally carries about 10 to fifteen pounds of nitrogen (N), 5 to 10 pounds of phosphorus, and 10 to 12 kilos of potassium consistent with ton. Poultry manure has a higher consciousness of these factors.

The National Organic Program (NOP) offers specific tips for the usage of manure. Composted manure is favored, however if uncooked manure is used, the timing of software program software is vital. When applying uncooked manure to land-developing flora for human consumption, it ought to now not be used inside one hundred twenty days of harvest for soil-touching appropriate for eating plant life or inner ninety days for non-soil-touching fit for human intake flowers.

Alfalfa Meal or Pellets: These comprise about three percent nitrogen and are normally used as animal feed. They are extraordinary fertilizer substances for excessive-price horticultural plant life but may be too pricey for area plant life. Alfalfa meal is notion to comprise increase factors that enhance its effectiveness as a delivery of plant vitamins.

Chapter 5: Propagation Methods For Fruit Plants

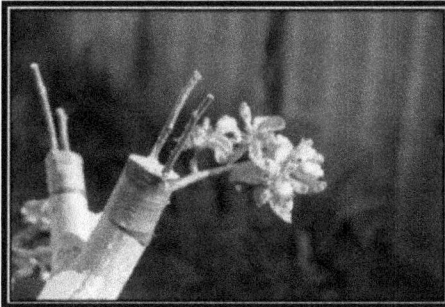

Saving seeds is a top notch exercising, and it's far honestly beneficial for every aspiring gardener to set up their very private seed bank. However, positive flowers and trees are better suitable for propagation. This is especially real for masses fruit bushes because the fruit super may not be as right as that of the figure plant. While it is beneficial to cultivate a whole lot of species and promote variety, it is commonly finest to make sure that the apple wooden you plant will yield scrumptious give up result.

Traditionally, human beings typically typically tend to go to nurseries to benefit younger sapling fruit timber, but this can be pretty expensive. On the alternative hand, propagating bushes is a price-powerful, thrilling, and without a doubt capability opportunity.

Exploring Seed Propagation and Grafting Techniques

Propagation Through Cuttings

Using cuttings for propagation is a fast method to establish new fruit trees. For instance, apple kinds can make bigger roots inner a month, and the cuttings may additionally already resemble small bushes. However, sure fruit tree cuttings require grafting onto a rootstock, which may not be cited here. These strategies are most suitable for fruit trees.

Note: Mediterranean quit end result like figs, pomegranates, mulberries, in addition to climbers together with grapes and kiwifruit, can all be cultivated from hardwood cuttings.

There are 3 forms of cuttings: softwood, semi-hardwood, and hardwood. Softwood cuttings are obtained from the bendy green stems within the course of spring and early summer season. The stems are appropriate for softwood cuttings after they'll be resultseasily snapped even as bent and feature younger leaves at the tip. Softwood cuttings root rapid, however precautions should be taken to prevent them from drying out.

Semi-hardwood cuttings are taken later in the one year at the same time as the inexperienced stems of the current year's increase have hardened and started to mature, generally in autumn. Although semi-hardwood cuttings take a bit longer to root, they'll be less at risk of drying out. Hardwood cuttings are obtained from mature dormant stems in late autumn, wintry weather, or early spring. Sometimes, hardwood cuttings are interested by a bit of the older department. Hardwood cuttings take an entire lot longer to propagate however require a good deal less attempt.

To prevent drying out, it's miles great to accumulate cuttings within the morning and plant them as soon as viable. If they want to be saved for some time, wrap them in moist paper towels or tissue. Collect robust, wholesome cuttings which is probably 4-6 inches (10-15 cm) lengthy. Remove the leaves from the lower one-zero.33 of the stem. When making prepared hardwood or semi-hardwood cuttings, make 1-2 inch (2.Five-five cm) slits thru the outer layer to beautify moisture absorption. Ensure that every one reducing gadget and pots are thoroughly wiped clean and preferably disinfected. Dip the stem in rooting hormone or willow water and insert it right proper right into a pre-made hole inside the soil.

The hole may be made in advance using a pencil or finger. Firmly % the soil and cover the cutting with a apparent plastic bag that has some holes for air float. Alternatively, an inverted jar or plastic bottle may be used. The motive is to hold excessive humidity and provide ok airflow. Opening or lifting the quilt as quickly as a day helps lessen the danger of mold and illnesses. Place the pot in oblique moderate at a temperature of 60-sixty 5 stages Fahrenheit (15-18 levels Celsius).

Using a heating mat set at 70 tiers Fahrenheit (21 degrees Celsius) will accelerate root development. Roots need to appear inner numerous months. Once an remarkable root device has shaped, transplant the slicing to a nutrient-rich soil. To save you rot, soil-a lot much less potting media in conjunction with perlite and sand are commonly used for rooting cuttings.

Using Potatoes For Propagation

A captivating technique employed thru advantageous gardeners includes a method to facilitate the growth in their very private rooted seedlings. To expedite and decorate the rooting method previous to planting in the soil mixture, cuttings are inserted into small potato tubers. Advocates of this approach argue that it offers additional vitamins to the cuttings, reduces moisture loss, and speeds up the formation of a root device, consequently making it simpler to propagate fruit timber.

To begin, pick out out the cuttings from the fruit bush you wish to plant. Firstly, take away all leaves about 1 inch (3cm) beneath the supposed ground degree for the shoot. Next, make a diagonal cut in some unspecified time in the future of the stem decreasing at a 45-degree mind-set. Subsequently, create a hollow in the potato this is genuinely huge enough to house the stem cutting securely.

Prepare your pot with the beneficial useful resource of putting round 2 inches (5cm) of soil at the lowest and characteristic the potato with the cutting on top. Finally, fill the pot with soil, and cover it with a plastic bag or glass jar. The preliminary sprouts will emerge inner a quick time frame.

Propagating From Seeds

Growing fruit trees from seeds is often considered time-consuming and every now and then even deemed not possible. However, on the same time as it is able to take some time for a seedling to come to be a mature fruit bush or tree, it might not take prolonged for it to turn out to be a small tree. The first step in seed propagation is accumulating the seeds. Most seeds are accrued in autumn. Many tree seeds require a length of bloodless and wet conditions before germination, referred to as stratification.

In nature, this happens at some stage in wintry weather whilst the seeds rest inside the soil, searching forward to spring. Therefore, the perfect manner to sow the seeds is in the fall, both out of doors in pots or on the ground in a shaded vicinity. Protect the seeds from hungry animals the usage of twine mesh or a cover. Alternatively, the herbal stratification technique may be simulated thru manner of chilling the seeds interior. To try this, soak the seeds in filtered water for forty eight hours, then place them in moist paper towels or sphagnum moss.

Store them in a area or bag in the refrigerator, ensuring the medium stays wet however not wet. Check on them after severa months to appearance inside the occasion that they have started to germinate. It's vital to word that many forestall end result grown from seeds will not produce the same shape of fruit as their figure tree. This is because of the reality give up end result at the side of apples, pears, and plums are frequently grafted onto a rootstock, and their seeds will not bring about the identical fruit range.

Propagation Using Willow Water

Willow water serves as a significantly powerful herbal rooting hormone for all sorts of plant cuttings. Additionally, it may be applied to water already installation flora, assisting in the development of robust root systems.

The mystery lies in Indolebutyric acid (IBA), a plant hormone responsible for stimulating root boom. Willow branches' developing hints consist of centered quantities of IBA. By extracting and soaking those lively sections of a willow branch in water, we will extract massive quantities of IBA that dissolve into the water.

Salicylic acid (SA), a chemical much like aspirin, is every other plant hormone determined in willow water. It plays a essential function in signaling a plant's protection mechanisms, specifically in the device called "systemic obtained resistance" (SAR). SAR triggers a plant's inner protection responses closer to pathogens even as one part of the plant is attacked, extending protection to various factors. Additionally, salicylic acid can purpose protection responses in nearby flora by manner of using remodeling into a volatile chemical compound.

When developing willow water, each salicylic acid and IBA are launched into the water, and each make contributions sincerely to the propagation of cuttings. Willow water, derived from the stems of the willow tree, acts as a herbal rooting hormone appropriate for cuttings and air layering. Its effectiveness stems from the presence of a particular hormone in willow timber that promotes root improvement, ensuing in rapid rooting of willow cuttings.

Willow water can be made at any time of the three hundred and sixty five days, despite the fact that spring is normally taken into consideration the top-exceptional season. To put together willow water, accumulate numerous cups of glowing willow twigs, making sure they will be no thicker than a pencil and approximately ½ inch thick. Select the most up to date, most present day, and greenest branches, cast off the leaves, and reduce them into small pieces, about 1 inch or three cm lengthy (smaller portions are fundamental). Place those reduce branches right into a bucket, big bottle, or any appropriate area, and cowl them with water. Allow the combination to take a seat down down for several days to four weeks.

Alternatively, you may steep the branches in boiling water for twenty-four-48 hours, this is a quicker method however does no longer yield as many rooted willow cuttings for future use. Once the aggregate has acquired a gel-like consistency or resembles prone tea, strain it the usage of a colander or sieve, keeping apart the willow portions from the liquid. Store the willow water in an hermetic jar, which can be refrigerated for up to 2 months. However, it's far more powerful even as used smooth.

Propagation Using Rooting Hormones

Raw honey: Some gardeners recommend that honey includes enzymes that might stimulate root increase in vegetation. Honey is likewise wealthy in nutrients B, PP, C, K, E, ascorbic acid, 35 minerals, and different elements. Additionally, its antibacterial and antifungal residences can be beneficial. Applying honey to the interface immediately or growing an answer with water are methods to use it. To make an answer, dissolve a teaspoon of honey in 1.Five liters of water. Dip the stem of the slicing into the answer and permit it soak for 12 hours.

Aloe vera: Aloe juice not great promotes root device improvement in cuttings however moreover strengthens the general immunity of destiny seedlings. Furthermore, aloe juice possesses antiseptic houses, efficiently disposing of risky microorganisms. To employ aloe vera, location 1 tablespoon of glowing aloe gel in a pitcher of water. Keep the cuttings immersed within the aloe water solution till root guidelines begin to emerge. This usually takes approximately per week.

Aspirin: When the usage of aspirin, opt for uncoated drugs and keep away from people with plastic coatings, due to the fact the plant does now not require those chemicals. Dissolve the pill in a pitcher of water and appearance beforehand to it to certainly dissolve. Then, area the cuttings within the water and permit them to soak for some hours to take in the aspirin solution.

Cinnamon: While cinnamon is not through and big a rooting hormone, it does have a beneficial effect on plant boom by means of manner of stopping fungal formation. This will boom the chance of the cuttings developing into wholesome fruit wooden. To employ cinnamon, sprinkle it on a plate or in a pitcher and lightly coat the lessen quit of the stem with the powder.

Apple cider vinegar: Another choice to save you fungal growth is apple cider vinegar. However, it is crucial to be cautious as excessive vinegar can harm the cuttings. Create an answer by means of using diluting a teaspoon of apple cider vinegar in 6 cups of water. Briefly dip the lowering into the solution after which plant it.

Propagation Through Air layering

Air layering is a manner of propagating wood in which a department is recommended to broaden roots at the identical time as though associated with the tree. It is just like floor layering but does no longer incorporate touch with the floor. Air layering is remarkable because of the reality it's miles quite smooth, appropriate for almost any tree type, and effects inside the growth of a high-quality fruit tree in a specifically brief time. There are not unusual strategies of air layering. The first method includes doing away with a hoop of bark from a suitable branch in which root formation is favored. The uncovered location is then included with sphagnum moss and wrapped with plastic to hold moisture.

Chapter 6: Planting And Establishing Fruit Trees

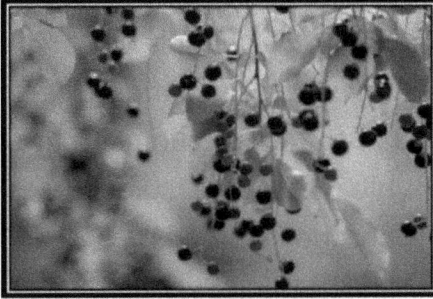

Knowing the proper method for planting fruit wooden is crucial to guarantee a thriving plant able to producing a bountiful harvest. Incorporating fruit wooden into your garden is an great idea, as they provide big delight. Whether it's far crisp apples or succulent plums, no longer has something compared to the delectable flavor of homegrown fruit, this is far extra energizing than what you may discover at the store.

Selecting Healthy Nursery Stock and Planting within the Right Season

Opt for the Smallest Tree: In business nurseries, trees regularly undergo severa styles of trauma, especially in the course of up-potting, that can result in tangled roots and a less-than-super situation. Therefore, it's far in reality useful to accumulate the smallest tree possible. By doing so, you lessen the period that the tree has spent on this potentially distressing surroundings, allowing it to spend more time flourishing within the nurturing embody of your garden. Personally, I discover the 5-gallon length to be the maximum crucial I choose to shop for, and I will pretty really select out a smaller length if it happens to be available.

Assess the Root Ball: Take the initiative to get rid of the basis ball from the pot yourself or are looking for assist from a knowledgeable staff member. While doing so, pay close to hobby to the circumstance of the roots. Are they tangled right right into a compact mass at the lowest of the pot? This may want to mean an damaging situation. Alternatively, did all the soil consequences fall off at the same time as the tree become taken out of the pot? In such instances, the tree has no longer but firmly installed its roots within the field. Ideally, you have to search for roots that maintain the soil together, with quality the rims of the pot revealing their presence.

Consider the Girth: It is critical to shift your consciousness away from the height of the tree, as you may likely need to trim off numerous toes while planting it. Instead, direct your hobby to the girth of the trunk. A thicker trunk suggests an advanced and sturdy tree, making it an awesome preference if to be had.

Evaluate Staking: Take a 2d to look at the manner the tree is tied to a stake. If the ties are excessively tight, it may advise a weaker trunk structure. Nurseries frequently strong bushes to stakes to encourage vertical increase, probably diverting strength faraway from growing a robust trunk. Additionally, test the shape of the trunk itself. Does it resemble a uniform pencil, with consistent thickness from pinnacle to bottom? In assessment, search for a trunk that famous power and possesses a sluggish taper, turning into thicker within the direction of the lowest.

Watch for Disease: Remain vigilant for any crucial signs and symptoms of essential ailment. Trees restrained to pots also can show off yellowing foliage due to their limited growth conditions. Be searching out exceptional symptoms of disorder, together with spotted leaves, lifeless limbs, or splits inside the bark alongside the trunk.

Best Time to Plant Fruit Trees

The important element in fruit tree planting is ensuring that they acquire sufficient water and vitamins during the preliminary months, which highlights the significance of timing. The number one purpose is to facilitate the establishment of a strong root device in your new tree.

In regions with slight climates, it's far possible to plant fruit wooden and wooden starting in

November. This time-body gives them a few extra weeks to allow their roots to installation in advance than boom resumes. For regions like the South and Pacific Northwest, this period is appropriate for planting.

In the coldest regions, the most favorable time to plant naked-rooted timber is in the direction of the give up of wintry weather or the first half of of spring. This is even as the ground is now not frozen, making it less complex to dig, however earlier than new boom initiates. Promptly planting the bushes upon their arrival is critical, usually inside more than one days. However, if the outdoor situations are negative, it is possible to percent the roots with moist soil to boom this time-body.

It is recommended to seek recommendation from a tree nursery acquainted together with your location to achieve steerage on the final window for lifting and delivering young plant life, as well as the precise conditions on your location.

How to Plant Fruit Trees

When it involves planting fruit wooden, it's miles nicely really worth noting that numerous authentic fruit-tree providers provide moderately priced kits that embody essential devices collectively with stakes, ties, mulch mats, and more. Disregarding those objects in an try to save cash is a faulty technique, because it fails to take into account the prolonged-term advantages they offer.

Begin through digging a hole that reaches the depth of a spade and spans approximately three toes in width. Opting for a square-typical hollow in desire to a round one is maximum best because it stimulates the roots to increase into the encircling floor. Remember to keep the soil you have excavated either in a wheelbarrow or on a massive plastic sheet.

Next, include some inches of awesome lawn compost into the bottom of the hollow the use of a garden fork. Thoroughly blending the compost is essential to save you the tree's roots from encountering a sudden transition among the compost and the ordinary soil. Similarly, make sure that you mixture a few compost into the soil you have had been given eliminated.

While putting the bare-rooted tree within the center of the hollow, be aware of the marginally darker "watermark" at the tree's trunk. This indicator denotes the precise soil stage at the time of its preliminary boom. To make sure proper planting intensity, align this line with the soil surrounding the hole. If important, make modifications by means of using along with or getting rid of soil. It's properly properly worth noting that most fruit timber are grafted onto a rootstock, and the graft union need to usually stay above the floor.

After briefly getting rid of the tree, insert a strong timber stake multiple inches far from the hollow's middle, ideally on the component from which the winning wind originates. Use a mallet to firmly hammer the stake into the ground.

Carefully area the tree back into the hole, ensuring its proximity to the stake, and start refilling the hollow with the soil-and-compost aggregate across the roots. Gently p.C. The mixture the usage of your boots, taking care no longer to reason any harm to the touchy roots. Once the hollow is half-stuffed, boom the tree via way of an inch and then allow it to settle backtrack. This mild lifting and dropping motion aids in the soil's powerful distribution throughout the roots.

Once all the soil has been brought and firmly packed, fasten the tree to the stake using a tie. Leave sufficient room for the tree trunk to increase, however avoid immoderate looseness. Additionally, if animals pose a hazard, recall setting a protective tube throughout the trunk. At this degree, it's also beneficial to sprinkle a small amount of seaweed meal fertilizer across the bottom, located by protective it with a biodegradable hemp mat to suppress weed growth.

To save you the roots from drying out and to inspire in addition agreement of the soil, thoroughly water the area. This step is critical in making sure the a fulfillment reputation quo of your fruit tree.

Until the basis device of the tree attains a period equal to or extra than its private, the tree remains incredibly susceptible to the detrimental influences of environmental stressors. In the preliminary twelve months of boom, insufficient water and nutrient deliver can effortlessly bring about the lack of lifestyles of the tree. Hence, it is critical to make sure the tree gets enough watering, especially in the direction of arid weather situations.

Chapter 7: Planning Your Orchard

Embarking on the journey to installation your orchard is an thrilling task that needs careful attention and strategic making plans. The achievement of your orchard hinges on meticulous alternatives made within the preliminary stages, in particular in selecting the proper fruit timber on your region and designing a format that optimizes boom and productiveness. In this whole guide, we delve into the intricacies of making plans your orchard, ensuring that every step is a purposeful stride within the path of a thriving and fruitful panorama.

Selecting the Right Fruit Trees for Your Region

The first and arguably most crucial step in planning your orchard is selecting fruit wood tailored in your area's weather, soil conditions, and microclimate nuances. The kind of fruit tree kinds is large, and now not every tree will flourish in each environment. Understanding your place's particular tendencies is pivotal in curating a desire that guarantees healthy increase and sufficient yields.

Climate Considerations

Start with the aid of manner of the use of assessing your area's weather. Is it temperate, subtropical, or arid? Different fruit wood thrives in super climatic situations. For instance, apples and cherries desire cooler climates with terrific seasons, while citrus timber flourishes in subtropical environments. Investigate the chilling hours required for high quality fruit sorts, as this performs a crucial role in the tree's dormancy and subsequent fruiting.

Soil Analysis

Conduct an in depth assessment of your soil. Fruit bushes have various soil alternatives, with factors which includes pH, drainage, and nutrient content material fabric cloth influencing their regularly taking place fitness. Apples and pears, as an example, usually select out properly-worn-out soils with a barely acidic to neutral pH. Stone fruits, like peaches and plums, frequently thrive in slightly acidic to independent soils with wonderful drainage. Understanding your soil's composition allows you to make knowledgeable alternatives about soil amendments and ensures the lengthy-term electricity of your orchard.

Microclimate Assessment

Consider the microclimates within your orchard web web page. Microclimates, prompted by using manner of factors which encompass slope, proximity to our bodies of water, and wind patterns, can drastically impact the success of specific fruit wooden. For example, sheltered regions may be perfect for frost-sensitive types, at the same time as prolonged places might be suitable for give up end result that benefit from expanded air drift. By figuring out and leveraging those microclimates, you optimize the conditions for each tree, fostering a resilient and thriving orchard.

Local Pest and Disease Resistance

Explore fruit tree sorts recognized for their resistance to famous pests and ailments to your vicinity. This proactive method can mitigate the need for excessive chemical interventions, aligning with sustainable and environmentally conscious orcharding practices. Local agricultural extension workplaces and horticultural societies frequently offer precious insights into the extremely good illness-resistant kinds, ensuring an improved and resilient orchard.

Designing Your Orchard Layout

With the choice of appropriate fruit wood tailor-made for your vicinity, the following segment of making plans involves designing a thoughtful format that maximizes daylight hours exposure, optimizes pollination, and helps inexperienced orchard manage. A properly-designed format is not nice aesthetically captivating but additionally serves because of the fact the blueprint for a harmonious and effective orchard.

Sunlight Optimization

Sunlight is the lifeblood of fruit manufacturing, and your orchard format need to prioritize maximizing daylight exposure for every tree. Consider the orientation of rows and the spacing amongst wooden to lessen shading. Generally, north-to-south row orientation is desired, ensuring that each tree gets adequate sunlight hours in the direction of the day. Adequate spacing among rows prevents overcrowding and permits for gold favored slight penetration to the lower branches.

Pollination Dynamics

Many fruit timber rely on pollination for fruit set, making the affiliation of properly ideal sorts a important interest to your orchard format. Group trees with comparable bloom instances and like minded pollination requirements to facilitate pass-pollination.

This intentional grouping complements fruit set, resulting in more strong harvests. Be aware of capacity cross-pollination barriers, together with bodily obstructions or versions in bloom timing, that might impact the efficacy of pollination.

Topography and Water Management

The herbal contours of your orchard web page, also called topography, play a pivotal feature in water manage. Consider the slope of the land to plan for proper drainage and prevent waterlogging, which can be destructive to fruit tree roots. Implement contour planting on slopes to restrict soil erosion and optimize water absorption. Additionally, layout swales or berms to direct water glide in which wanted, making sure green irrigation and lowering the hazard of water-related stress on your wood.

Windbreak Considerations

Wind may have each excellent and lousy effects on fruit timber. While mild breezes useful resource in pollination and discourage high-quality pests, strong winds can damage blossoms and more youthful fruit. Strategically planting windbreaks, which incorporates shrubs or trees, on the windward side of your orchard gives safety without compromising air glide.

This considerate format element safeguards your fruit timber from capability wind damage, contributing to a more resilient orchard surroundings.

Accessibility and Orchard Maintenance

Practical issues for orchard management are in addition vital within the format format. Ensure that pathways and alleys are large enough to residence tool for planting, pruning, and harvesting. This now not first-class lets in ease of motion however additionally minimizes the chance of soil compaction round tree roots. Plan for storage regions for device and device, and keep in mind integrating composting stations to recycle herbal substances, fostering a sustainable technique to orchard renovation.

Cultivating the Blueprint for Success

In the problematic dance of making plans your orchard, the careful preference of fruit wooden and the considerate format of the orchard format are the cornerstones of success. It is a meticulous manner that dreams a harmonious aggregate of ecological attention, horticultural knowledge, and practical concerns. As you embark in this journey, envision now not certainly rows of timber but a dynamic and thriving surroundings-a testomony to the synergy among nature and the intentional efforts of the orchardist.

This whole manual serves as a compass, guiding you thru the nuanced selections that shape the destiny of your orchard. From know-how the proper wishes of every fruit variety to crafting a format that optimizes boom, every step is a sensible stride closer to a panorama teeming with the promise of blossoms and the anticipation of plentiful harvests. In the chapters that observe, we delve deeper into the seasonal care, protection, and the myriad intricacies that remodel a nicely-deliberate orchard right right into a flourishing testament to the artwork and technological expertise of fruit farming.

Chapter 8: Planting And Early Care

Embarking on the journey of planting and nurturing fruit wooden is just like laying the ideas of a thriving orchard. This important section demands a mixture of precision, care, and foresight to make certain the prolonged-time period health and productiveness of your wooden. In this comprehensive manual, we will delve into the nuances of getting began, protecting everything from proper tree planting techniques to the intricacies of initial pruning and training.

As we domesticate the tips, envision each tree as a promise- an investment that, with considerate care, will go through fruit for years to come.

Proper Tree Planting Techniques

The act of planting a fruit tree isn't a trifling placement of roots into soil; it is a ceremony that defines the tree's future. Proper tree planting techniques are foundational to the tree's hooked up order, influencing its increase, nutrient uptake, and fashionable resilience. Let's discover the important thing factors that make contributions to successful tree planting.

Site Selection and Soil Preparation

Before delving into the bodily act of planting, considerate website preference and soil education set the degree for fulfillment. Choose a domain with nicely-tired soil and enough daylight, retaining off low-lying regions prone to waterlogging. Conduct a soil check to assess pH and nutrient tiers, amending the soil as had to create an gold preferred surroundings for root improvement. Remove weeds and particles from the planting net web page to cast off competition for belongings.

Selection of Quality Trees

Investing in brilliant nursery wood is vital to a a success orchard. Choose wooden with nicely-superior root systems, free from symptoms of sickness or damage. Inspect the tree's trunk for a at once and strong shape, and make sure that the branches are lightly allocated. Healthy, lively nursery trees provide a strong start for your orchard, increasing the hazard of a fulfillment established order.

Planting Hole Preparation

The planting hole is the tree's gateway to the soil, and its schooling is a critical step inside the approach. Dig a hole this is wider than the tree's root ball and of sufficient depth to address the roots without bending or crowding. Create a slight mound of soil at the lowest of the hollow to help the tree's herbal root flare. The cause is to installation a solid and nicely-aerated surroundings that promotes wholesome root enlargement.

Planting Procedure

As you lower the tree into the planting hole, make sure that the foundation collar- the problem in which the roots meet the trunk- is level with the soil floor. To remove the air pocket, carefully tamp the earth as you backfill the hole. To assist the soil settle and the roots stay hydrated, deliver the tree hundreds of water. Apply a layer of mulch throughout the base of the tree, leaving a gap across the trunk to prevent moisture-associated troubles. Mulching aids in weed control, temperature regulation, and soil moisture conservation.

Staking and Support

While staking is not always vital, it could offer valuable help, specifically for more youthful or inclined wood. Use bendy ties to attach the tree to the stake, bearing in mind mild movement that encourages trunk electricity. Monitor the tree regularly to ensure that the ties do no longer grow to be too tight and preclude increase. As the tree establishes, frequently lessen staking and allow it to broaden its natural power.

Watering Regimen

Establishing a consistent watering routine is crucial within the early degrees of tree planting. Young bushes are particularly vulnerable to drought strain, and making sure an desirable sufficient and regular water deliver is important for root development. Water deeply and normally, adjusting the frequency based totally on weather conditions. A drip irrigation system or a watering basin across the tree's base can facilitate green and focused watering.

Initial Pruning and Training

Beyond the act of planting, the initial pruning and training of fruit wood are pivotal steps which have an impact on their shape, shape, and destiny productivity. Pruning is an paintings that consists of strategic removal of branches to encourage crucial increase, beautify air go with the flow, and shape the tree for accessibility and harvesting. Let's delve into the crucial factor standards and strategies of preliminary pruning and education.

Pruning Goals and Timing

The overarching aim of pruning is to installation a properly-balanced and open cover that allows daylight hours penetration and air go with the flow. The timing of pruning is based upon on the sort of fruit tree and nearby climate. Generally, dormant season pruning- executed at some point of past due wintry weather or early spring earlier than new growth emerges- is favored for max fruit wooden. This timing minimizes stress on the tree and permits for maximum pleasing restoration of pruning wounds.

Structural Pruning for Form and Balance

Structural pruning focuses on shaping the tree's commonplace shape and inspiring a strong scaffold form. Remove any competing or crossing branches, aiming for nicely-spaced limbs that radiate outward from the most important trunk.

Identify the imperative leader-the principle vertical stem-and ensure its dominance to sell upward increase. Encourage lateral branches that form massive angles with the trunk, as those are an entire lot much less susceptible to breakage.

Training Young Trees: Espalier and Central Leader Systems

The desire of schooling gadget is predicated upon on the kind of fruit tree and the popular orchard layout. Espalier, a tool that consists of schooling wood to increase in a flat, -dimensional form in the course of a aid shape, is right for constrained place and can be visually attractive.

The applicable leader tool, in which a single, dominant vertical stem is advocated, is commonplace for lots fruit wooden, together with apples and pears. Consider the long-term desires of your orchard and choose out out a schooling device that aligns in conjunction with your imaginative and prescient.

Renewal Pruning for Health and Longevity

Renewal pruning consists of the periodic removal of older wood to stimulate the increase of recent, active shoots. This exercising rejuvenates the tree, keeps its productiveness, and opens up the cover for sunlight hours penetration. Identify and cast off any lifeless, diseased, or willing wooden for the duration of renewal pruning. Pay hobby to the general stability of the tree, aiming to create a cowl that permits daytime to attain all elements of the tree.

Disease Prevention and Pruning Tools

Pruning device play a vital characteristic in achieving easy cuts and minimizing stress at the tree. Ensure that your pruning device are sharp and nicely-maintained to avoid tearing or crushing branches. Before transferring from tree to tree, disinfect your device to save you the unfold of sicknesses.

Pruning is likewise an possibility to test out the tree for signs and signs and symptoms of pests or ailments, contemplating early intervention and manipulate.

Pruning Challenges and Common Mistakes

While pruning is a precious capacity, it can present traumatic situations, specially for beginners. Common mistakes include over pruning, that would strain the tree and decrease fruiting capability, and wrong cuts that depart stubs or damage the department collar.

Striking a balance among conducting pruning dreams and respecting the tree's natural boom behavior is crucial. Regular statement and adjustment of pruning practices based totally definitely at the tree's response contribute to ongoing fulfillment.

As you navigate the realms of planting and early deal with your fruit timber, envision every step as a gesture of willpower to the destiny. From the first-class act of planting, which establishes the tree's connection to the soil, to the artistry of pruning, which shapes its shape and productivity, each desire is a brushstroke inside the canvas of your orchard.

Through considerate care, strategic making plans, and an expertise of the precise desires of every tree, you aren't just cultivating an orchard; you're nurturing the promise of seasons to return. The orchard's infancy is a touchy but transformative phase, and with every passing one year, your wood will stand as a testomony to the understanding and care invested of their earliest days.

Chapter 9: Nurturing Healthy Growth

The adventure of cultivating a fruitful orchard is a non-stop partnership many of the orchardist and the timber, each diploma requiring considerate attention and strategic care. As we delve into the arena of nurturing healthful growth, we navigate the intricacies of soil schooling and fertilization, and discover the nuanced practices of watering fruit bushes.

This holistic technique to orchard care lays the foundation for a resilient and thriving environment, in which the roots of healthy growth increase deep into the soil and branches attain for the sky.

Soil Preparation and Fertilization

A thriving orchard starts offevolved with the soil underneath your wood- an complicated surroundings that serves as the inspiration for healthy boom. Soil education and fertilization aren't clearly obligations; they may be dynamic techniques that require a keen facts of the soil's composition, nutrient dreams, and the symbiotic courting among roots and earth.

Soil Testing: Unveiling the Soil's Secrets

Before embarking on any soil steerage or fertilization routine, behavior an entire soil take a look at to clear up the mysteries underneath the surface. Soil trying out offers treasured insights into the soil's pH, nutrient stages, and texture, empowering you to tailor your approach primarily based surely at the best traits of your orchard. Laboratories or agricultural extension services will have a observe soil samples, presenting hints for unique amendments and fertilization strategies.

Soil pH Adjustment: Creating an Optimal Environment

The soil pH diploma has a big impact on how without problems accessible nutrients are to fruit trees. The pH range that maximum timber choose is barely acidic to impartial. Lime is normally used to elevate pH in acidic soils, at the identical time as elemental sulfur can decrease pH in alkaline soils. Adjusting soil pH ensures that important vitamins are in a form that wood can and no longer the use of a trouble absorb, selling wholesome boom and nutrient uptake.

Organic Matter and Soil Structure Enhancement

Incorporating natural rely wide variety range into the soil enhances its form and fertility. Well-rotted compost, aged manure, or cover flowers contribute natural fabric, improving soil texture, water retention, and nutrient-maintaining capability. This natural enrichment fosters a great environment for microbial hobby, growing a thriving soil ecosystem that lets in the health of fruit tree roots.

Strategic Fertilization: Meeting Nutrient Demands

Fertilization is a touchy dance that involves presenting critical vitamins within the proper proportions and on the right instances. The three primary vitamins- nitrogen, phosphorus, and potassium- play excellent roles in fruit tree fitness. Nitrogen promotes leafy boom, phosphorus permits root improvement and flowering, at the equal time as potassium contributes to everyday strength and fruit exceptional. Specialty fertilizers formulated for fruit timber often consist of micronutrients like zinc and boron, addressing unique needs for maximum growth.

The timing of fertilizer software application is crucial. In widespread, fruit wooden gain from a balanced fertilizer finished in past due winter or early spring before new growth begins. Avoid excessive nitrogen in past due summer season or fall, as it can stimulate overdue-season boom that can be susceptible to wintry climate damage.

Watering Practices for Fruit Trees

Water, the elixir of lifestyles, is a valuable useful resource in orchard care, and reading effective watering practices is fundamental to keeping healthful boom. Fruit timber have particular water requirements, and imparting regular moisture within the proper portions guarantees strong root development, good enough nutrient uptake, and time-honored electricity.

Understanding Water Needs: Tailoring to Tree Requirements

The water desires of fruit bushes evolve throughout the growing season, caused through way of elements which incorporates tree age, weather conditions, and soil type. Newly planted wood require ordinary watering to installation their root structures, whilst mature bushes benefit from deep, infrequent watering to encourage deep root increase. Understanding the moisture alternatives of your precise fruit tree sorts allows you to tailor your watering practices for this reason.

Deep Watering vs. Surface Irrigation: Encouraging Root Depth

Encourage deep root increase by education deep watering in desire to common surface irrigation. Deep watering turns on tree roots to boom into the soil, enhancing their functionality to get proper of get admission to to vitamins and resist periods of drought. Drip irrigation systems, soaker hoses, or watering basins across the tree's drip line are powerful strategies for turning in water right away to the basis place. Minimize overhead watering to reduce the risk of foliage illnesses and ensure green water utilization.

Mulching: Conserving Moisture and Regulating Temperature

Mulching is a multitasking ally in orchard care, imparting advantages that amplify past moisture conservation. A layer of natural mulch, inclusive of wooden chips or straw, serves as a shielding blanket for the soil, lowering evaporation, suppressing weeds, and moderating soil temperature. Mulching also mitigates soil compaction, a common problem in orchards, via manner of imparting a buffer amongst heavy rain or irrigation and the soil floor.

Monitoring Soil Moisture: Precision in Irrigation

Regularly display soil moisture to notable-tune your irrigation practices. The use of soil moisture sensors or manual inspection of soil situations allows you to gauge at the same time as and what form of water your fruit trees want. Adjust irrigation schedules based totally on weather patterns, incorporating herbal rainfall into your calculations. Overwatering can result in root suffocation and nutrient leaching, even as underwatering can also moreover result in strain, decreased boom, and compromised fruit incredible.

Seasonal Adjustments: Adapting to Nature's Rhythms

Recognize the seasonal fluctuations in water necessities and adapt your watering practices as a end result. During durations of energetic increase, inclusive of spring and early summer time, fruit wood have higher water needs. Adjust irrigation frequency and duration to meet the ones increased dreams. Conversely, reduce watering in late summer time and fall as trees put together for dormancy. Observing and responding to the natural rhythms of your orchard fosters a dynamic and responsive technique to water manipulate.

In the complicated dance of nurturing wholesome increase, soil preparation, and fertilization, and watering practices emerge as the choreography that sustains the power of your orchard. Every motion is a test within the symphony of growth, from the high-quality amendments to the soil that lay the inspiration for sturdy roots, to the clever software software of water that quenches the thirst of blossoming branches.

As you traverse the seasons for your orchard care, envision every tree as a testomony to the thoughtful orchestration of these practices- an embodiment of the partnership between your stewardship and the natural elements.

By cultivating deep facts of your orchard's precise wishes and responding with care and precision, you nurture not simply timber however a thriving surroundings in which the roots of healthy boom run deep and the branches reap for the promise of fruitful seasons in advance.

Chapter 10: Seasonal Care And Maintenance

Cultivating a thriving orchard is a harmonious interaction many of the diligent orchardist and the ever-converting seasons. Each level, from the spring awakening of blossoms and pollination to the summer time vigilance over foliage, thinning, and pests, and in the long run, the fall training encompassing harvesting and winterization, demands a nuanced technique.

In this complete manual, we embark on a journey thru the seasons, unveiling the secrets and techniques and techniques and strategies of seasonal care and protection that loose up the whole functionality of your orchard.

Spring Awakening: Blossoms and Pollination

Blossom Inspection and Bud Break

As wintry climate's hold close loosens, the orchard undergoes a paranormal transformation in spring. The first order of enterprise is to analyze blossoms and observe bud harm. This visible evaluation serves as a fitness check for the timber. Monitor buds for any signs and symptoms and signs and symptoms of wintry weather damage and examine the general electricity of each tree. Timing of bud spoil varies amongst fruit tree types, and know-how this transformation enables in gauging the overall fitness of your orchard.

Pollination Strategies

Spring is the season of romance for fruit bushes, where the touchy dance of pollination happens. Understanding the pollination requirements of your orchard is paramount. Ensure that pollinators like bees are energetic at a few degree inside the blooming duration. For self-pollinating bushes, the presence of pollinators can decorate common fruit production. Consider planting pollinator-first-class flora or introducing beehives to create an environment conducive to a fulfillment pollination.

Thinning for Optimal Fruit Set

Following a success pollination, the subsequent strategic circulate is thinning. Thinning consists of the selective removal of extra stop result to allow the closing ones to get maintain of sufficient nutrients and sunlight. It may additionally moreover seem counterintuitive to get rid of potential culmination, but thinning prevents overcrowding, complements fruit length, and reduces the hazard of branches breaking underneath the burden of an excessive fruit load.

Fertilization Adjustments

Spring is a crucial time for a second round of fertilization. Actively growing wood have accelerated dietary needs, and adjusting your fertilization technique is crucial. Utilize soil check results to tailor your technique to an appropriate dreams of your orchard. A balanced, slow-launch fertilizer can provide sustained vitamins at some point of the developing season. The application expenses must be adjusted based totally on factors like tree age, length, and widespread fitness.

Summer Vigilance: Foliage, Thinning, and Pests

Monitoring Foliage and Nutrient Levels

Summer brings forth the colorful foliage that sustains the orchard's engine of boom. Regular monitoring of leaves is vital to come to be privy to symptoms of nutrient deficiencies, pest harm, or illnesses. Addressing troubles proper away guarantees the general fitness of the orchard. Adjust nutrient ranges based totally on visual assessments and, if essential, greater soil finding out to provide most useful useful resource throughout this period of active photosynthesis.

Thinning Continued: Strategic Adjustments

The thinning approach initiated in spring may additionally additionally require extra interest in early summer season. Evaluate the final fruit clusters and thin similarly if wanted. Focus on maintaining regular spacing among give up end result and doing away with any misshapen or damaged specimens. Thinning ensures that the strength of the tree is directed in the route of fewer culmination, resulting in massive, healthier specimens at harvest.

Pest and Disease Management

Summer is a season of heightened pest interest, demanding vigilant pest control techniques. Regularly take a look at bushes for signs and symptoms of pests at the side of aphids, mites, and caterpillars. Implement protected pest control (IPM) practices, which may encompass introducing beneficial insects, utilizing horticultural oils or insecticidal soaps, and the use of cultural practices like pruning to limit pest habitat.

Disease manipulate is similarly critical. Fungal sicknesses, collectively with apple scab and powdery mould, thrive in warmness, humid conditions. Implement preventative measures like utilising fungicides regular with a schedule, making sure right spacing among wood for air motion, and eliminating infected plant fabric. Timely disease control safeguards the overall fitness of the orchard.

Irrigation Optimization

Fine-tune your irrigation practices to meet the increasing water desires of actively developing timber and growing fruit. Adjust watering schedules primarily based totally mostly on climate conditions, contemplating rainfall and temperature fluctuations. Deep, uncommon watering encourages strong root increase and decreases the hazard of floor root improvement, that could make wooden prone to drought stress.

Fall Preparation: Harvesting and Winterization

Harvest Timing: Precision and Flavor

As summer season gracefully offers manner to fall, the orchard reaches a crescendo with the graduation of the harvest. The timing of the harvest is a delicate balance among engaging in final ripeness and stopping overripening at the tree. Familiarize yourself with the particular harvest home windows for every fruit range to your orchard. Factors together with shade, firmness, and taste imply readiness. Harvesting in tiers allows for most fine fruit tremendous and minimizes waste.

Post-Harvest Care: Cleanup and Pruning

After the final fruit has been plucked, it is time for placed up-harvest care. Remove any fallen fruit to reduce the chance of pests and illnesses overwintering within the orchard. Conduct a thorough cleanup, getting rid of debris and weeds. Fall is likewise an opportune time for pruning. Identify and cast off useless or diseased branches, and form the tree for most useful form. Pruning in fall promotes wound recovery and prepares the tree for wintry weather dormancy.

Winterization: Protecting Against the Cold

As the temperatures drop and wintry weather strategies, winterization measures come to be vital. Protect younger or inclined trees from wintry weather sunscald by means of the usage of wrapping the trunks with tree wraps. Apply a layer of mulch throughout the bottom of the wooden to insulate the soil and defend roots from freezing temperatures. In regions with immoderate winters, remember burlap or defensive coverings to guard wood from harsh situations.

Tool Maintenance and Planning for the Next Season

The wintry weather months provide an possibility for tool protection and coaching for the imminent season. Clean and sharpen pruning tool to make sure unique cuts. Take inventory of additives and order any crucial materials for the following season. Use this time for instructional hobbies, staying informed approximately the modern orchard control strategies and upgrades.

Orchestrating Success Through the Seasons

In the complex symphony of seasonal care and protection, every word done via using the orchardist contributes to the grand crescendo of a thriving and fruitful orchard. From the touchy blossoms of spring to the vigilant care of summer time and the meticulous arrangements of fall, the adventure thru the seasons is a non-stop rhythm of increase, nurturing, and stewardship.

As you embark on this orchard odyssey, recall that success lies now not truly in person obligations but inside the seamless integration of seasonal practices. Through energy of mind, information, and a deep reference to your orchard, you grow to be the conductor of an orchestra wherein each tree, each blossom, and each fruit play its particular detail within the perennial melody of increase and abundance.

Chapter 11: Managing Pests And Diseases

Cultivating a thriving orchard is a touchy dance with nature, and one of the key worrying conditions on this ballet is the manager of pests and illnesses. In this entire manual, we are capable of delve into the intricacies of identifying commonplace issues that afflict fruit timber and find out herbal pest control strategies. By understanding the nuances of these worrying conditions and embracing sustainable solutions, you could foster a healthy and resilient orchard environment.

Identifying Common Issues

Signs of Pest Infestation

Early detection of pest infestations is crucial for effective control. Regularly investigate your fruit timber for signs and signs of pests, which could encompass:

Visible Damage: Look for chewed or broken leaves, end end result with holes, or bark harm. These are commonplace signs of pest presence.

Excrement or Residue: Pests often depart in the returned of droppings, webbing, or particular residue. Examine leaves and branches for such signs and symptoms and symptoms.

Distorted Growth: Abnormal increase styles, collectively with twisted or stunted branches, may additionally moreover signal the presence of pests.

Wilting or Discoloration: Yellowing or wilting leaves may be a symptom of severa issues, which include pest infestation.

Recognizing Common Pests

Different pests pose unique demanding situations to fruit wood. Familiarize your self with commonplace orchard pests:

Aphids: Small, gentle-bodied insects that suck sap from leaves and stems, inflicting distortion and yellowing.

Scale Insects: Often decided on branches, the ones pests seem as small, flat, or domed systems. They feed on plant juices.

Caterpillars: Larvae of moths or butterflies that eat foliage, culmination, or buds.

Spider Mites: Microscopic arachnids that feed on plant juices, inflicting stippling and leaf discoloration.

Fruit Flies: These bugs lay eggs in ripening fruit, and their larvae purpose fruit damage.

Detecting Common Diseases

Diseases also can compromise the fitness of fruit bushes. Watch for the ones common troubles:

Fire Blight: A bacterial illness that reasons wilting, blackening, and a scorched look in branches, just like fireplace damage.

Apple Scab: A fungal ailment resulting in darkish lesions on leaves and fruit, leading to defoliation.

Powdery Mildew: A fungal infection characterised by way of the use of a powdery white substance on leaves, affecting photosynthesis.

Brown Rot: A fungal illness inflicting brown, rotting spots on stop end result, especially common in stone fruit.

Citrus Canker: A bacterial infection inflicting lesions on leaves, fruit, and stems in citrus trees.

Organic Pest Control Methods

Companion Planting

Strategic planting of partner vegetation can assist deter pests. Consider integrating the subsequent:

Marigolds: Their heady scent repels nematodes and some bugs.

Basil: Acts as a natural insect repellent and complements the taste of neighboring vegetation.

Nasturtiums: Attract aphids a long way from awesome flora, serving as sacrificial hosts.

Beneficial Insects

Encourage natural predators that feed on dangerous pests. Introduce or entice useful insects which include:

Ladybugs: Consume aphids and one-of-a-kind soft-bodied pests.

Parasitic Wasps: Lay eggs on caterpillars or insect eggs, controlling their populations.

Predatory Beetles: Feed on numerous pests, which includes aphids and mites.

Neem Oil

Derived from the neem tree, neem oil is an organic answer with insecticidal houses. It serves as an insect repellant and messes with the pest's life cycle.

Application: Dilute neem oil ordinary with package commands and study as a foliar spray.

Frequency: Apply frequently, especially at some stage in the developing season or whilst pests are most energetic.

Diatomaceous Earth

Consisting of fossilized diatoms, diatomaceous earth is a herbal insecticide that damages the exoskeleton of insects.

Application: Sprinkle a thin layer on the soil or straight away on flowers susceptible to crawling pests.

Caution: Use warning to avoid inhalation, as diatomaceous earth may be an irritant.

Garlic Spray

Garlic has natural insect-repelling homes. Garlic spray may be powerful within the route of quite a few pests.

Homemade Solution: Mix overwhelmed garlic cloves with water, permit it steep, and strain earlier than spraying.

Coverage: Ensure thorough coverage, in particular at the undersides of leaves wherein pests regularly hide.

Kaolin Clay

Kaolin clay paperwork a defensive barrier on plant surfaces, deterring pests and lowering disorder incidence.

Spray Application: Mix kaolin clay with water and spray on leaves, growing a white movie.

Reflective Properties: The reflective floor might also moreover confuse and repel pests, reducing feeding.

Chapter 12: Harvesting The Bounty

The culmination of months of care and cultivation, the harvest season in an orchard is a second of satisfaction and pleasure for any fruit grower. Knowing even as to achieve and employing right harvesting techniques are pivotal steps that could notably impact the first-rate and flavor of the cease end result you've got labored so diligently to domesticate.

In this comprehensive guide, we're able to find out the nuances of harvesting, from facts the symptoms of readiness to the use of techniques that make sure a bountiful and flavorful yield.

Knowing When to Harvest

Color as a Key Indicator

One of the primary visible cues indicating fruit readiness is its colour. The transformation of inexperienced to the fruit's function hue signs ripeness. However, it's far essential to recognize that the right colour can vary amongst fruit sorts.

Apples: Look for a exchange in color from inexperienced to the apple's function hue (purple, yellow, or a mixture).

Peaches and Nectarines: A ancient past coloration shift from green to yellow shows ripeness.

Plums and Cherries: A deepening of color and a moderate offer to touch endorse readiness.

Citrus Fruits: Citrus types regularly turn from green to yellow or orange, counting on the type.

Firmness and Texture

The texture of the fruit can offer precious insights into its readiness for harvest.

Apples and Pears: Press gently close to the stem. If the fruit yields barely and separates with out problem, it's miles in all likelihood ripe.

Peaches, Nectarines, and Plums: A slight squeeze need to bring about a moderate supply without being overly moderate.

Berries: Ripe berries are plump, juicy, and effects detach from the stem or plant.

Citrus Fruits: Feel for a employer but barely yielding texture even as lightly squeezing the fruit.

Aroma and Fragrance

The aroma emanating from the fruit can be a sensory clue to its ripeness.

Peaches and Nectarines: A candy fragrance close to the stem suggests ripeness.

Melons: A fruity aroma on the blossom quit indicates readiness.

Apples: A subtle, fruity heady scent close to the stem shows ripeness.

Berries: Fragrance is often greater cited at the same time as berries are absolutely ripe.

Taste and Flavor Development

While taste is the final test of ripeness, it might not be possible to sample each fruit.

Sample a Few: Select a representative sample of end result and taste-test them to gauge time-venerated ripeness.

Follow the Harvest Window: Familiarize your self with the usual harvest window for each fruit variety to ensure most awesome flavor.

Proper Harvesting Techniques

Use the Right Tools

Equipping yourself with the perfect device guarantees a smooth and inexperienced harvest.

Pruning Shears: Ideal for reducing stems and branches without inflicting harm.

Harvesting Knife: Suitable for culmination with thicker stems or those requiring precise cuts.

Fruit Picking Pole: Extends your attain for cease end result excessive in the tree, which consist of apples or pears.

Handheld Clippers: Useful for smaller branches and fruits, providing precision.

Harvest inside the Morning

Early morning is regularly the most amazing time for harvesting end quit end result.

Cool Temperatures: Cooler temperatures help hold the fruit's freshness inside the route of harvesting.

Reduced Pest Activity: Insects and pests are commonly an awful lot much less active inside the morning.

Optimal Sugar Content: Sugar content material cloth is regularly maximum within the morning, contributing to higher taste.

Handle with Care

Gentle managing at some point of harvesting prevents bruising and harm to the end result.

Avoid Dropping: Place end result gently on your harvesting area to prevent bruising.

Handle with Clean Hands: Wash your arms in advance than harvesting to keep away from shifting dust or contaminants.

Use Soft Containers: Go for bins that won't purpose abrasions or harm to delicate fruits.

Harvesting Specific Fruits

Different culmination have unique trends that require particular harvesting strategies.

Apples and Pears: Twist the fruit slightly on the equal time as lifting to detach it from the spur. Alternatively, use a moderate upward movement while handpicking.

Peaches and Nectarines: Hold the fruit lightly and twist, permitting the herbal separation from the tree.

Plums: Twist the fruit gently or use pruning shears for large branches.

Berries: Use your fingertips to gently pluck ripe berries, leaving the stem intact.

Citrus Fruits: Use pruning shears to lessen the stem, leaving a small thing connected to the fruit.

Storage Considerations

Proper storage is essential to retaining the exquisite of harvested cease result.

Temperature and Humidity: Store stop result at the tremendous temperature and humidity stages for every range.

Ventilated Containers: Use containers that permit for air flow to save you moisture buildup.

Check for Ripeness: Regularly check stored cease end result for ripeness and remove any overripe or broken ones.

Harvesting the Fruits of Your Labor

Harvesting is the crescendo in the symphony of fruit cultivation, a second while the cease stop end result of your efforts is realized within the bounty of your orchard.

By studying the art work of recognizing at the same time as to collect and using right harvesting techniques, you make certain that the end result of your tough artwork are not only ample however furthermore of the tremendous excellent.

As you embark on every harvest season, bear in mind it a celebration of the partnership amongst you and your orchard. Each cautiously decided on fruit is a testomony for your dedication, understanding, and the herbal rhythms of the bushes.

May your harvest be ample, your culmination flavorful, and your orchard a supply of pride and delight.

Chapter 13: Preserving And Enjoying Your Harvest

The pride of a bountiful harvest extends some distance beyond the instant of selecting ripe end end result from the branches. To recognize the flavors of your orchard at some point of the seasons, gaining knowledge of the artwork of safety is crucial.

In this complete manual, we will discover the techniques of canning, freezing, and drying give up end result, making sure that the abundance of your harvest may be loved prolonged after the wood have shed their leaves. Additionally, we are going to dive into scrumptious recipes and culinary pointers that elevate your preserved stop give up end result into culinary delights.

Canning Fruits for Long-Term Enjoyment

Materials Needed for Canning

Jars with Lids: Choose jars appropriate for canning, making sure they will be freed from cracks or chips.

Canning Equipment: This consists of a water bath canner for immoderate-acid give up end end result and a stress canner for low-acid cease result.

Fruit Preparation Tools: Peelers, corers, and slicers for inexperienced fruit steering.

Acid Additives: Lemon juice or citric acid may be had to maintain color and taste.

Canning Methods

Water Bath Canning: Suitable for excessive-acid forestall end result like berries, peaches, and tomatoes. Submerge sealed jars in boiling water to create a vacuum seal.

Pressure Canning: Necessary for low-acid stop result like apples, pears, and plums. The better temperatures ensure the elimination of micro organism.

Step-thru-Step Canning Process

Prepare the Jars: Sterilize jars and lids with the resource of immersing them in boiling water. Ensure they will be very well dry earlier than use.

Prepare the Fruit: Wash, peel, center, and slice the fruit as desired.

Fill the Jars: Pack organized fruit into sterilized jars, leaving adequate headspace.

Add Acid: For fine fruits liable to discoloration, upload lemon juice or citric acid to keep colour and taste.

Prepare Syrup or Liquid: Depending at the fruit, prepare a syrup or liquid to pour over the fruit inside the jars.

Remove Air Bubbles: Run a non-metallic utensil along the inner of the jar to release any trapped air.

Wipe Jar Rims: Ensure the jar rims are smooth and dry in advance than setting the lids.

Secure Lids: Place sterilized lids on the jars and regular them with metal bands.

Process in Canner: Follow the proper canning method (water bath or stress canning) and technique the jars for the preferred time.

Cool and Test Seals: Allow jars to loosen up, and take a look at seals through the use of pressing down on the middle of each lid. A well sealed lid want to not pop once more.

Label and Store: Put a date and contents label on each jar earlier than storing it. Store in a fab, dark location.

Freezing Fruits for Freshness

Preparation Steps for Freezing

Clean and Prepare: Wash and prepare the fruit, removing pits, cores, or stems.

Blanch Certain Fruits: Blanching allows hold colour, taste, and dietary price. It includes in quick immersing quit result in boiling water, accompanied thru a right away ice tub.

Dry Thoroughly: Ensure fruits are thoroughly dried to prevent ice crystals and freezer burn.

Packaging: Use airtight bins, freezer luggage, or vacuum-sealed luggage for packaging.

Fruits Suitable for Freezing

Berries: Strawberries, blueberries, raspberries.

Stone Fruits: Peaches, plums, apricots.

Citrus Segments: Freeze citrus segments for a sparkling addition to liquids or desserts.

Bananas: Peel and slice bananas for smoothies or frozen treats.

Tips for Freezing Success

Flash Freezing: Spread forestall quit end result on a baking sheet for preliminary freezing before shifting to packing containers. This prevents clumping.

Avoid Overpacking: Leave a few room in packing containers for end result to extend as they freeze.

Label Containers: Clearly label boxes with the fruit type and date.

Use Freezer-Friendly Containers: Choose packing containers designed for freezer use to prevent freezer burn.

Drying Fruits for Concentrated Flavor

Methods of Drying

Sun Drying: Traditional approach regarding publicity to the solar. Appropriate for climates with low humidity.

Dehydrator: Controlled drying with an electric powered dehydrator, suitable for some of cease result.

Oven Drying: Use a low oven placing to slowly dry give up result.

Fruits Suitable for Drying

Apples: Slice into jewelry or chips.

Grapes: Become raisins whilst dried.

Apricots and Peaches: Slice for solar-drying or dehydrating.

Bananas: Create banana chips.

Steps for Drying Fruits

Prepare the Fruit: Wash and slice end cease end result lightly for uniform drying.

Pre-Treatment: Some end cease end result advantage from pre-remedy to maintain color and save you oxidation. Options encompass dipping in lemon juice or blanching.

Arrange on Drying Trays: Arrange fruit slices in a single layer on drying trays, ensuring proper air bypass.

Drying Process: Follow the unique commands for your preferred drying method. Sun drying also can take numerous days, at the equal time as a dehydrator can expedite the device.

Check for Dryness: Fruits should be pliable however now not sticky. Check for dryness with the resource of pressing the center of a slice; it ought to not be moist.

Cooling Period: Allow dried end result to kick back in advance than packaging.

Packaging: Store in hermetic boxes or vacuum-sealed luggage.

Delicious Recipes and Culinary Tips

Preserved Fruit Compote

Ingredients:

2 cups blended preserved give up quit end result (peaches, plums, berries)

1/4 cup honey or maple syrup

1 teaspoon vanilla extract

1 cinnamon stick

Zest of one orange

Instructions:

Combine preserved give up cease result, honey or maple syrup, vanilla extract, cinnamon stick, and orange zest in a saucepan.

Simmer over medium heat until the aggregate thickens and flavors meld.

Remove the cinnamon stick in advance than serving.

Serve the compote warmth over yogurt, ice cream, or as a topping for pancakes.

Frozen Fruit Smoothie Bowl

Ingredients:

1 cup frozen combined berries

1 frozen banana, sliced

half cup Greek yogurt

1/4 cup almond milk

Toppings: easy berries, sliced almonds, granola, and chia seeds,

Instructions:

In a blender, combine frozen berries, frozen banana, Greek yogurt, and almond milk.

Blend until smooth and creamy.

Pour the smoothie right right into a bowl.

Top with smooth berries, sliced almonds, granola, and chia seeds,

Enjoy a sparkling and nutritious smoothie bowl.

Dried Fruit and Nut Energy Bites

Ingredients:

1 cup blended dried give up end result (apricots, apples, raisins)

1 cup nuts (almonds, walnuts, or a aggregate)

1/4 cup nut butter (almond butter, peanut butter)

1 tablespoon honey

half of teaspoon cinnamon

Shredded coconut for coating (non-compulsory)

Instructions:

In a meals processor, combine dried stop end result, nuts, nut butter, honey, and cinnamon.

Pulse the mixture until a sticky dough is shaped.

Roll the combination into small electricity bites.

Optional: Roll the bites in shredded coconut for introduced texture.

Refrigerate for as a minimum half of of an hour prior to serving.

These energy bites make a handy and nutritious snack.

Preserving and gambling your harvest is a journey that extends the orchard's bounty a long way beyond its branches. Whether you choose the undying manner of lifestyles of canning, the benefit of freezing, or the centered flavors of drying, every technique lets in you to satisfaction in the essence of your orchard all through the converting seasons.

As you embark at the culinary journey of the use of preserved cease end result, the recipes and hints provided provide a glimpse into the diverse tactics you could growth your dishes. From colourful fruit compotes to smooth smoothie bowls and healthful strength bites, your preserved culmination become key elements in a symphony of flavors that satisfaction the senses.

May your pantry be full of jars of preserved delights, your freezer stocked with end result prepared for mixing, and your kitchen infused with the engaging aroma of dried culmination. With every chunk, get delight from now not just the taste but the end end result of your efforts, turning a harvest into a tapestry of culinary creations that celebrate the richness of every season.

Chapter 14: Troubleshooting And Problem-Solving

Cultivating a flourishing orchard is a worthwhile employer, but it comes with its percent of disturbing situations. From pests and illnesses to environmental elements, orchardists regularly find themselves coping with limitations that require activate attention and strategic answers.

In this complete guide, we can delve into troubleshooting commonplace disturbing situations in orchards, imparting professional advice and problem-solving techniques to make sure the health and energy of your fruit-bearing haven.

Dealing with Common Challenges

Pest Infestations

Challenge: Aphids, mites, caterpillars, and one of a kind pests can threaten the health of your fruit wood.

Expert Advice:

Integrated Pest Management (IPM): Implement a holistic method that mixes organic, cultural, and chemical controls. This also can consist of introducing useful bugs, the use of insecticidal soaps, and training suitable orchard hygiene.

Regular Monitoring: Inspect your wooden regularly for symptoms of pests. Early detection reduces the opportunity of damages and allows activate intervention.

Companion Planting: Strategically plant partner plants that repel pests. Marigolds, as an instance, can deter nematodes, while basil acts as a herbal insect repellent.

Diseases Impacting Trees

Challenge: Fungal, bacterial, and viral ailments, alongside side apple scab, fireplace blight, and powdery mildew, can compromise the general health of your orchard.

Expert Advice:

Proactive Measures: Adopt preventative strategies, which include right spacing among timber for air go with the flow, making use of fungicides or bactericides as encouraged, and deciding on sickness-resistant sorts.

Pruning Practices: Prune wooden to inspire airflow and sunlight hours penetration, reducing the conditions conducive to fungal illnesses.

Sanitation: Remove and break infected plant material right away to prevent the spread of illnesses.

Soil Issues and Nutrient Deficiencies

Challenge: Soil that lacks essential nutrients or has an wrong pH can stop tree increase and fruit development.

Expert Advice:

Soil Testing: Perform everyday soil tests to decide nutrient ranges and pH. Adjustments can then be made based totally on the precise desires of your orchard.

Fertilization Strategy: Develop a tailored fertilization plan considering the nutritional necessities of your fruit bushes. Organic amendments, together with compost, can decorate soil shape and fertility.

Mulching: Apply natural mulch throughout the bottom of timber to keep moisture, suppress weeds, and frequently growth the soil because it breaks down.

Environmental Stressors

Challenge: Adverse climate conditions, alongside aspect frost, drought, or immoderate warm temperature, can strain wooden and impact fruit manufacturing.

Expert Advice:

Frost Protection: Employ frost protection measures, which include using frost fabric or applying water to create a defensive ice layer. Site preference and planting frost-resistant sorts additionally play a role.

Drought Mitigation: Implement efficient irrigation practices, which includes deep watering to encourage deep root growth. Mulching allows maintain soil moisture throughout dry durations.

Heat Stress Management: Provide color at some point of intense warmness occasions, specifically for younger or susceptible trees. Proper pruning also can beautify airflow, reducing warm temperature stress.

Poor Fruit Development or Small Harvests

Challenge: Trees may additionally produce fewer or smaller end result due to different factors, together with terrible pollination, inadequate nutrients, or wrong pruning.

Expert Advice:

Pollination Enhancement: Encourage pollinators, together with bees, by way of the use of planting pollinator-first-rate flowers and averting excessive use of insecticides in the path of bloom.

Thinning Fruits: Overcrowded cease give up result can result in smaller sizes. Practice thinning to allow good enough spacing, enhancing the dimensions and tremendous of the remaining give up end result.

Adjust Fertilization: Fine-track your fertilization approach primarily based totally on tree requirements. Excessive nitrogen, for instance, can result in active vegetative growth at the fee of fruit development.

Expert Advice for Overcoming Issues

Consult Local Agricultural Extension Services

Expert Advice:

Local Expertise: Seek steering from community agricultural extension offerings or horticultural professionals acquainted with the specific traumatic situations of your location.

Soil Testing Services: Many extension offerings offer soil trying out offerings, offering targeted insights into your soil's composition and nutrient stages.

Educational Resources: Take benefit of workshops, seminars, and academic materials supplied via extension services to live informed about the modern-day orchard manipulate practices.

Professional Arborist or Horticulturist Consultation

Expert Advice:

Diagnostic Expertise: If worrying conditions persist, keep in mind consulting with a professional arborist or horticulturist. Their diagnostic expertise can pick out out nuanced issues.

Tree Health Assessment: Professionals can confirm common tree fitness, discover pressure factors, and endorse focused interventions.

Tailored Recommendations: Receive custom designed tips primarily based absolutely totally on the ideal situations of your orchard, ensuring a customized technique to hassle-solving.

Network with Fellow Orchardists

Expert Advice:

Community Resources: Join neighborhood orchardist corporations, on line boards, or community agencies wherein reviews and solutions are shared.

Peer Experiences: Learn from the memories of fellow orchardists who also can have confronted similar annoying situations. Peer insights can offer precious perspectives.

Collaborative Problem-Solving: Engage in collaborative trouble-fixing, sharing your annoying conditions and searching out enter from others who've correctly navigated comparable situations.

Nurturing a Resilient Orchard

In the tapestry of orchard control, stressful conditions are inevitable, but with strategic trouble-solving and professional recommendation, you may nurture a resilient and thriving orchard. By addressing commonplace troubles which embody pests, illnesses, soil deficiencies, and environmental stressors, you no longer most effective guard the fitness of your trees however moreover optimize fruit production.

Remember that each orchard is unique, and a tailored approach to troubleshooting is essential. Utilize close by information, visit professionals even as wanted, and tap into the collective understanding of fellow orchardists. In the dynamic adventure of orchard cultivation, your dedication to proactive problem-solving ensures that your orchard no longer most effective survives traumatic situations however flourishes with resilience and electricity.

Chapter 15: Choosing The Right Fruit Tree

Container gardening flourishes on the concept of optimizing restricted area without compromising on the pleasure of nurturing plants. In this segment, we'll delve into the clean enchantment of compact-sized fruit bushes, usually called dwarf bushes, and how they flawlessly align with the thoughts of field gardening. Growing organic fruit wood in boxes is a likely choice for human beings with constrained area or who want more manages over the developing conditions. It allows you to revel in the benefits of fruit timber at the equal time as accommodating smaller yards, balconies, or patios. Selecting the proper fruit tree range is important in your subject orchard adventure. Dwarf and semi- dwarf types offer unique advantages which could impact the achievement of your mini orchard. Dwarf fruit timber flawlessly fuses nature's splendor and flexibility to human desires. Their compact period, early adulthood, and generous yields motive them to satisfactory partners for those looking for the amusing of fruit tree cultivation in restrained areas. As we discover similarly, you'll find out the processes to harness the functionality of dwarf wooden to create a thriving and efficient discipline orchard, all on the identical time as reveling in the magic of those botanical wonders. The connection with nature frequently feels remote in the coronary heart of bustling cities. Yet, the enchantment of compact-sized fruit bushes gives city dwellers a extremely good possibility to bridge this hole. Dwarf wood serve as gateways, allowing town residents to forge a substantial reference to nature at their doorstep. Compact fruit trees are the architects of transformation, turning omitted corners

UNDERSTANDING DWARF TREES

Dwarf fruit wooden are testaments to human ingenuity and nature's variability. The partnership among grafting strategies, genetic mutations, and boom- regulating factors outcomes in their fascinating compactness. By unraveling this complex dance among technological knowledge and nature, you'll recognize the artistry that has crafted those miniature wonders, allowing you to hold the magic of orchards into the maximum compact areas. The union of scion and rootstock is a testament to the artistry of horticulture, providing a international of opportunities for compact fruit timber that deliver the pleasure of orchards into the smallest city regions. Dwarf and semi-dwarf fruit wood are cultivated kinds which have been selectively bred or grafted to provide smaller, extra compact wood. These smaller timber are well-known among home gardeners and orchard growers who want greater area or need to make fruit harvesting and renovation more feasible. Dwarf fruit bushes usually attain a peak of 6 to eight toes (1.Eight to two.Four meters), while semi-dwarf timber can grow barely taller, sporting out spherical 10 to twelve toes (3 to 3.7 meters). Standard fruit timber can develop up to 20-5 toes (7.6 meters). Despite their smaller period, dwarf and semi-dwarf fruit wooden can though produce massive fruit. They commonly start bearing fruit at an earlier age in comparison to traditional-sized timber. Since the tree is smaller, accomplishing the fruit for harvesting, pruning, and pest manage is greater ability. Dwarf and semi-dwarf fruit wooden are commonly properly-tailor-made to severa climates and can be grown in areas wherein their fashionable contrary numbers ought to likely battle. They are regularly greater cold-hardy and may withstand cooler temperatures. The decreased period of dwarf and semi-dwarf wooden is achieved thru grafting them onto rootstocks that truely restrict their growth. Rootstocks are decided on primarily based totally on contamination resistance, energy, and compatibility with the popular fruit range. Pruning dwarf and semi-dwarf wood are extra to be had due to their smaller

THE LITTLE ORCHARD THAT COULD

size. They require plenty a great deal less location for boom, and pruning enables keep their form, manipulate length, and sell higher fruiting. These wooden are frequently much less complicated to spray, net, and guard in competition to pests and sicknesses. Rootstocks make contributions to the dimensions manage of compact fruit wooden and serve as guardians, arming these trees in competition to the challenges of drought and soil-borne conditions. By tapping into their fantastic potential to optimize water utilization and sell disease resistance, rootstocks play a pivotal characteristic in making sure the survival and prosperity of your mini orchard. Rootstocks with drought tolerance and illness resistance characteristic the unsung heroes of compact fruit wooden, fostering an environment of health, resilience, and sturdiness. The synergy amongst those abilities ensures that your mini orchard now not most effective endures but flourishes, weathering demanding conditions and growing more potent with time. As we development, you'll find out techniques to harness those skills to cultivate a flourishing, enduring discipline orchard that could be a testament to the harmonious dance between nature and human stewardship.

Remember that even as dwarf and semi-dwarf bushes offer many benefits, they will have barely reduced power in assessment to conventional-sized timber. Adequate watering, fertilizing, and pest control care are important to ensure healthy boom and best fruit production. Before shopping any fruit tree, it's advocated to research the perfect necessities and trends of the range you're inquisitive about and any close by hints or problems from nurseries to your place.

SELF-POLLINATION

Self-pollination is a first rate botanical phenomenon perfect for compact fruit tree cultivation. Understanding its significance empowers you to harness the self-enough reproductive competencies of those wooden, making sure that your mini orchard flourishes with healthful, considerable, and delicious fruit. Self- pollination in fruit wood refers back to the machine in which the plant life of a single tree can pollinate themselves and produce fruit without requiring the transfer of pollen from each other tree. In self-pollinating fruit timber, the plant life comprise every male (stamens) and woman (pistils) reproductive organs. The pollen from the stamens is transferred to the stigma of the equal flower or a new stigma

within the same tree. This can upward thrust up via herbal techniques like wind, vibrations, or all movements or with the assist of pollinators including bees or one in every of a kind bugs. Several fruit tree species are recounted for their self-pollinating trends and emerge as saviors of compact orchards, supplying a sensible and green method to the worrying conditions of circulate-pollination in limited areas. By putting off the need for multiple tree plantings, those flexible bushes redefine the possibilities of fruitful cultivation in city and small-scale settings. Let me located it this manner. If you've got sorts of fruit timber that aren't self-pollinating, you will need 4 and only styles of fruit. If you've got

got had been given self-pollinating fruit timber, you could get extra one-of-a-type ones and have 4 varieties of fruit. Now, that's a touch orchard that could.

However, checking the specific pollination requirements of the fruit tree range you would love to broaden is continuously advocated, as not all cultivars interior a species may be self-pollinating. When deciding on self-pollinating fruit timber for planting in containers, it is critical to consider types which are properly- appropriate to box gardening and function compact growth conduct. Here are a few self-pollinating fruit tree options that might thrive in packing containers:

Self-Pollinating Apple Trees

Dorsett Golden': A dwarf apple tree that produces yellow, crisp apples

Cox's Orange Pippin': A compact apple tree with sweet and fragrant fruit.

Jonagold': A semi-dwarf apple tree with large, candy-tart apples.

Self-Pollinating Peach Trees

Bonanza': A compact peach tree that produces juicy, yellow-fleshed fruit.

Stark Saturn': A dwarf peach tree with first rate taste and appealing freestone peaches.

Golden Jubilee': A semi-dwarf peach tree with massive, yellow peaches

Self-Pollinating Cherry Trees

Stella': A compact cherry tree that produces sweet, darkish pink cherries.

Compact Stella': Like Stella' however with a more compact growth dependancy.

THE LITTLE ORCHARD THAT COULD

Black Gold': A semi-dwarf cherry tree with agency, black cherries.

Self-Pollinating Plum Trees

Santa Rosa': A famous plum tree with candy and juicy reddish-crimson fruit.

Methley': A compact plum tree that bears sweet, reddish-skinned fruit.

Beauty': A semi-dwarf plum tree that produces large, candy plums.

Self-Pollinating Citrus Trees

Meyer Lemon': A small, evergreen tree with fragrant, juicy lemons.

Calamondin': A compact citrus tree with small, sour oranges frequently used for ornamental capabilities.

Kaffir Lime': A small lime tree identified for its fragrant leaves and specific- regular fruit.

Recently, I preferred to strive growing Calamondin and Meyer Lemon. They produced fruit the number one twelve months, even as I must want to wait about years to deliver fruit with a regular fruit tree. These are only some examples, and certainly one of a kind self-pollinating fruit wooden are also suitable for field gardening. When choosing fruit timber, consider the mature tree's length, the rootstock it's far grafted onto (which influences its last length), and the weather necessities of the precise range. Be sure to provide ok daylight, regular watering, and suitable care to ensure the health and productivity of your potted fruit timber.

GROW ZONES FOR FRUIT TREES

Grow zones are geographic areas with specific weather situations. The success of your compact fruit tree orchard hinges for your expertise of the network weather and the correct situations that impact plant boom. They manual your choices and strategies for cultivating fruit trees in restrained regions. In the sector of horticulture, information the idea of develop zones is like unlocking a map to a success gardening. This phase sheds mild on the definition of increase zones and their pivotal function in guiding your selections and techniques for cultivating fruit wooden, mainly in compact orchards. When developing fruit timber in containers, the concept of boom zones or hardiness zones however applies, no matter the truth that there are a few extra worries to do not forget. Here's how develop zones relate to fruit wooden in bins:

Start with the useful resource of figuring out fruit tree sorts endorsed to your unique hardiness location. This will assist ensure that the tree is customized to the same old temperature kind of your area. Lucky for you, developing fruit timber in containers affords some flexibility in accommodating unique hardiness zones. Containers may be moved indoors or to sheltered locations inside the direction of durations of bloodless or heat, permitting you to create microclimates that could enlarge the proper sort of fruit tree sorts. Containers offer the gain of manipulating microclimates more efficiently and fast than ones planted within the ground. Placing boxes in numerous places or adjusting their position can create microclimates that offer foremost conditions for precise fruit tree kinds. For instance, allow's say you live in zones 3 or four, and you need to expand citrus fruit; however the reality that citrus fruit is produced greater inside the southern states, in containers, you can skip your wood indoors or a greenhouse in which you create a microclimate defensive them from the cruel winters.

Protecting container-grown fruit timber from freezing temperatures is vital in regions with much less heat climates. Insulating the packing containers with bubble wrap, hessian sacks, or blankets in the course of wintry weather can assist save you the roots from freezing. Moving the boxes to a protected location or indoors throughout freezing periods additionally can be beneficial at the same time as deciding on packing containers for fruit wood.

These select sizes accommodate the tree's root gadget and increase conduct. Adequate box length lets in for correct root improvement and prevents the tree from turning into root-sure. This is specially essential for making sure the tree can resist temperature extremes in its specific hardiness zone. Containers are greater prone to temperature fluctuations than wooden planted in the ground. During excessive bloodless or warm temperature intervals, the temperature round the sector responds to defend the wood. This can also encompass providing color, mulching the soil floor, or watering to slight temperature swings. Ensure that the packing containers have true drainage to save you waterlogged soil, that would bring about root rot, and you don't want

THE LITTLE ORCHARD THAT COULD

that. Well-draining soil and enough field drainage holes are essential for keeping healthy root structures. Container-grown fruit timber may additionally moreover require greater frequent watering than in-ground ones, so show soil moisture tiers and regulate watering because of this. Similarly, alternate fertilization practices to satisfy the nutritional needs of the trees in bins, as the soil amount and nutrient availability may additionally additionally differ from in-floor plantings. Don't fear; I will bypass into greater detail approximately a number of these gadgets later.

The suitability of severa cease result for specific develop zones is predicated upon on severa elements, collectively with temperature, frost tolerance, chilling necessities, and warmth tolerance. Here are some examples of fruits and their famous suitability for first-rate growing zones:

Apples (Malus domestica): Apples may be grown in a large style of growing zones, with precise varieties suitable for special zones. Many apple sorts require numerous chilling hours within the path of winter to break dormancy and bring fruit. Some popular apple types for precise expand zones encompass Gala' (Zones 4-nine), Honeycrisp' (Zones 3-8), and Granny Smith' (Zones 8-eleven).

Citrus Fruits (e.G., oranges, lemons, limes): Citrus give up end result thrive in warmer climates. They are usually grown in USDA Zones Sep 11 or regions with slight winters. Examples consist of Washington Navel Orange' (Zones Sep 11), Eureka Lemon' (Zones 9-11), and Key Lime' (Zones 9-11).

Strawberries: Strawberries are flexible and may be grown in a giant form of expand zones. Different sorts have diverse levels of cold tolerance. Some well-known strawberry kinds embody June-bearing' sorts like Seascape' (Zones four-eight) and Everbearing' kinds like Albion' (Zones 4-eight).

Blueberries: Blueberries have unique soil and weather requirements. They pick out acidic soil and cooler climates. Common blueberry types appropriate for unique make bigger zones include Blue crop' (Zones 4-7), Jersey' (Zones 4-8), and Misty' (Zones five-10).

Peaches: Peaches thrive in areas with warm summers and slight winters. They are normally grown in Zones 5-8, no matter the truth that a few sorts are suitable for Zones four and nine. Popular peach kinds encompass Red Haven' (Zones five-8), Elberta' (Zones 5-nine), and Belle of Georgia' (Zones 5-eight).

Cherries: Cherries have great types appropriate for developing zones.

Sweet cherries require a wonderful huge variety of chilling hours, on the identical time as sour cherries are more cold-hardy. Examples embody Bing' candy cherry (Zones 5-8), Montmorency' sour cherry (Zones 4-7), and Stella' sweet cherry (Zones 5-9). It is essential to word that these hints are fashionable hints, and particular microclimates interior every develop area may have an effect on fruit tree achievement. It is constantly useful to go to expert gardeners for your location for extra specific hints primarily based completely for your vicinity. Here is a photograph of the develop zones that will help you higher understand. For the ones of you who are seen novices and recognize topics arms-on, like me, this could assist hundreds.

CHILL HOURS

Chill hours, additionally referred to as chilling hours or chilling gadgets, are utilized in horticulture and agriculture to quantify the bloodless exposure wanted for positive plant life, mainly fruit timber, to interrupt dormancy and resume not unusual boom

and improvement.

THE LITTLE ORCHARD THAT COULD

During wintry weather, deciduous fruit timber go through a period of dormancy to shield themselves from freezing temperatures. This dormant duration is crucial for his or her survival and healthful boom. This is on the same time as you may need to transport your fruit tree outdoors for them to get right sit down again hours till you preserve your own home this cold otherwise you stay in an igloo. Chill hours are accrued at or under a specific temperature range inside this dormant period. Chill hours are calculated thru recording the quantity of hours a fruit tree is uncovered to temperatures among a wonderful diploma, typically 32°F (zero°C) and forty five°F (7°C). These temperatures are taken into consideration superior for chilling requirements for max deciduous fruit tree types. Different fruit tree kinds have specific chilling necessities and vary based totally clearly on the tree's species, type, and geographic starting. Some fruit trees require fewer loosen up hours, even as others need greater to interrupt dormancy and initiate not unusual growth in spring. Chilling hours acquire at some stage in the wintry climate, because of this each hour spent indoors the correct temperature range adds to the entire loosen up hours. For example, if a fruit tree tales five hours at forty°F and three hours at 35°F, the entire collected sit down once more hours might be eight. Adequate sit down lower again hours are essential for fruit timber to boom and bring a healthful crop because of the truth insufficient loosen up hours can motive now not on time bud ruin, reduced flowering, or negative fruit set. Conversely, excessive relax hours may additionally additionally cause early bud damage, advanced susceptibility to overdue frost harm, or erratic increase styles. The variety of take a seat again hours required and the usual wintry weather temperatures variety in the course of precise areas and climates. Areas with milder winters may also need to don't forget the particular sit down decrease returned hour necessities of fruit tree kinds suitable on your place. It is nicely well worth noting that whilst sit down again hours are a vital hobby for fruit tree preference, they may be not the handiest hassle. Other factors like warmth requirements, pollination desires, soil type, and sickness resistance have to additionally be considered at the same time as deciding on fruit tree kinds for your precise place.Top of Form Chill hours but play a position in the boom and improvement of fruit bushes in packing containers, however the dynamics can be barely high-quality in evaluation to bushes planted inside the ground. Here are some vital factors regarding sit back hours and fruit wooden in boxes. Fruit tree sorts suitable for your region and hardiness area

want to nonetheless be decided on, thinking about their chilling necessities. Look for self-pollinating or low-relax variety sorts for in-field gardening. These sorts are generally extra adaptable to diverse take a seat back hour situations. The chilling hours professional via potted fruit bushes may additionally moreover range from those within the floor. Potted timber may also moreover enjoy slightly exceptional microclimates than wood planted within the garden due to discipline material, duration, and area. The proximity to partitions or houses can affect temperature fluctuations in the course of the field. Keep tune of the close by climate conditions and display your area's accumulation of sit back hours. Use weather critiques or consult neighborhood agricultural extension offerings for common loosen up hour information. However, it is important to be aware that those values are normally based totally on ground-planted timber, so the actual kick back hours professional thru potted trees might also range. Containers can offer a few diploma of insulation, affecting the take a seat lower back hour accumulation. Smaller pots can also revel in extra terrific temperature fluctuations than larger ones. Consider presenting more protection, together with wrapping the pots with insulating materials, in the course of extra freezing days to maintain extra solid temperatures. Potted fruit trees can occasionally experience earlier bud smash in comparison to floor-planted wooden because of the warmer situations furnished with the useful resource of containers. This early bud ruin can also moreover surrender stop result from an accelerated capability to past due frost occasions. Be prepared to protect the growing buds and flora at some point of temperature drops by the use of in brief overlaying the tree or transferring it to a sheltered place. Regularly test the boom and improvement of your potted fruit timber within the course of the wintry climate months. Look for signs and signs of bud swelling or distinct warning symptoms of the cease of dormancy. This will help you verify the development and determine while to transition the tree from dormant to lively increase thru adjusting temperature or watering.

While take a seat decrease lower back hours are essential, specific elements which encompass daylight hours, watering, soil amazing, and fertilization are further important for potted fruit timber' commonplace fitness and productivity. You can help your potted fruit trees thrive and convey a a achievement harvest via supplying gold general care and creating favorable growing situations.

The chilling hour requirements vary notably among wonderful fruit tree species and sorts. So here's a preferred assessment of the approximate

THE LITTLE ORCHARD THAT COULD

take a seat down again hour necessities for a few commonplace fruit tree kinds:

Apples: Apple bushes have numerous chilling necessities depending on the range. Apple wood require numerous 800 to at least one,500 chill hours. However, low-loosen up apple varieties require as low as three hundred to 500 lighten up hours.

Peaches: Peach wooden have mild to immoderate chilling necessities. Most peach sorts require round six hundred to 900 sit down back hours, in spite of the truth that some low-loosen up kinds can tolerate as few as 250 to four hundred relax hours.

Cherries: Cherry trees have a considerable sort of chilling necessities. Sweet cherries usually want a higher massive type of relax hours, starting from 800 to as a minimum one,2 hundred hours, on the identical time as bitter or tart cherry kinds have lower requirements, usually spherical four hundred to 800 loosen up hours.

Plums: Plum timber have mild chilling requirements. Most plum types require 500 to 900 take a seat down again hours, notwithstanding the reality that some low-chill plum sorts are available that want as few as 200 to 4 hundred sit back hours.

Pears: Pear trees commonly have moderate to immoderate chilling requirements. European pear types usually require around six hundred to at the least one,000 loosen up hours, while a few Asian pear types could have decrease requirements, beginning from 3 hundred to 600 relax hours.

Citrus: Citrus bushes, inclusive of oranges, lemons, and limes, have low chilling necessities compared to deciduous fruit timber. Most citrus timber need only one hundred to three hundred sit down once more hours. However, they may have unique temperature necessities sooner or later of the wintry climate to make sure maximum efficient fruit improvement. Re- member that those are substantial recommendations, and the take a seat down once more hour requirements may moreover range amongst unique cultivars internal each fruit tree kind. Researching and choosing sorts nicely-suitable to your area's weather and commonplace take a seat down lower again hour accumulation is critical. Consulting professional growers to your region can offer treasured insights into the particular relax hour requirements for the fruit tree types you need to domesticate. To summarize this segment about sit down returned hours, fruit trees want to be bloodless for a certain quantity of time so as for them to come out of dormancy and produce a bud that will become fruit. Now that you recognize all about dwarf wooden, the developing zones and hardiness of each, zones for the extremely good fruit wooden, and the distinction among self-pollinating and fruit trees that want a mate to endure fruit, you may now pick out the sort of

Chapter 16: From The Ground Up

Beneath the ground of your compact orchard lies a worldwide of life and sustenance—the soil. In this financial ruin, we'll delve into soil's importance in fruit tree cultivation. From its composition to its effect on root health, you'll find out how expertise and being concerned on your soil can bring about flourishing timber and bountiful harvests. The soil beneath your compact orchard is a treasure trove of vitamins, microorganisms, and existence-giving houses that right away impact the fitness and productivity of your fruit wood. By appreciating the elaborate relationship between soil and tree growth, you can create an surroundings that nurtures roots, fosters energy, and yields an abundance of delectable harvests, which incorporates DIY recipes, to assist maximize the increase of your fruit tree. In the beyond, even as you attempted to increase plants or fruit wooden, how plenty significance did you supply soil or fertilizer? When I have become knee-excessive to a grasshopper, I continuously concept you without a doubt placed the timber in the floor, and that become it. Dad taught me this lesson with the resource of letting me plant and evaluate my trees to what he produced. His trees commonly grew more sizable and with greater fruit, and it simply taught me how vital the right soil combination is to fruit bushes.

THE IMPORTANCE OF SOIL

Soil is important in plant growth and the overall fitness of discipline fruit wood. To prevent the ache of getting to analyze this as I did, I'm going to tell you a few

key motives why soil is crucial for fruit trees grown in packing containers:

Fruit wooden require a balanced supply of nutrients to thrive and bring wholesome quit result. The soil in containers must be rich in critical nutrients like nitrogen, phosphorus, potassium, and micronutrients. They orchestrate the increase and energy of your fruit timber. Good-great soil offers those vitamins to the tree roots, making sure right boom and fruit improvement. The soil in packing containers have to have the potential to preserve proper enough moisture for the fruit tree roots whilst moreover permitting more water to drain away. It need to stability water retention and drainage to save you overwatering or waterlogging, that can bring about root rot and excellent problems. Fruit timber in packing containers have limited place for root boom in comparison to the ones planted within the ground, so the soil want to provide a appropriate surroundings for root improvement, permitting the roots to spread and installation a healthful root machine. This facilitates the tree anchor itself and soak up vitamins correctly. The pH diploma of the soil influences nutrient availability to flora. Different fruit tree species have precise pH requirements for optimum perfect increase and fruit production. The soil in containers can be tested and changed to maintain the suitable pH variety for the fruit tree range. It ought to have an amazing shape that allows air to gain the roots. Adequate aeration prevents the roots from turning into waterlogged and promotes wholesome root respiratory. It also permits beneficial soil microorganisms to thrive, helping nutrient cycling and standard soil fitness. Healthy soil can make contributions to ailment and pest resistance in fruit bushes. Well-draining soil with proper natural rely content cloth can help save you the improvement of fungal infections and discourage dangerous pests.

Additionally, the presence of organisms can beautify natural pest manage mechanisms. The soil in boxes offers stability to the fruit tree, stopping it from toppling over and appearing as an anchor, preserving it upright and stable. When developing fruit timber in containers, it's far important to select out a wonderful potting mixture or create a suitable soil mixture that meets an appropriate desires of the tree species. Regular tracking of soil moisture, fertility, pH levels, and suitable watering and fertilization are important to maintain primary soil conditions for fruit wood' boom and productiveness.

THE LITTLE ORCHARD THAT COULD

CHOOSING THE RIGHT SOIL

Beneath the floor of your compact orchard lies a critical choice as a way to shape the destiny of your fruit timber—the selection of soil. By records the intricacies of soil preference, you'll set the quantity for a thriving mini orchard on the way to flourish for years. When selecting soil for fruit trees in boxes, it's miles important to don't forget their unique desires and requirements. Here are some factors to remember whilst deciding on a suitable soil.

Fruit timber choose properly-draining soil to save you soggy conditions leading to root rot. Look for a soil combo with appropriate drainage homes, allowing extra water to go with the float freely via the world's drainage holes. While it is important for the soil to empty nicely, it want to furthermore have the capability to hold moisture. Fruit wood want normal moisture levels to thrive. Choose a soil mixture that could maintain enough water to maintain the roots effectively hydrated with out becoming waterlogged. Fruit wood have specific nutrient requirements to aid their boom and fruit manufacturing, so pick a nutrient-wealthy soil blend that can launch nutrients efficiently. Adding compost or natural count number to the soil can decorate its nutrient content material. Different fruit tree species have numerous pH opportunities. Some decide upon slightly acidic soil (pH beneath 7), on the identical time as others thrive in impartial to slightly alkaline soil (pH above 7). Consider the pH requirements of your precise fruit tree and pick out out a soil blend that aligns with those needs. Adjusting the pH If important, the pH can be changed, like sulfur or lime. Container-grown fruit trees gain from a mild-weight soil mixture that is simple to deal with and promotes accurate airflow to the roots. Avoid heavy clay soils that may compact resultseasily and restriction right root boom, so search for a mixture that consists of herbal depend like peat moss, coconut coir, or perlite, which lets in decorate soil shape and aeration. Choosing a immoderate- incredible potting combination or growing your soil combination with sterilized components can assist reduce the threat of introducing pests, diseases, or weed seeds into the arena. Sterilized soil reduces the opportunities of problems arising from pathogens and undesirable plants. Consider the sector length you suggest to apply in your fruit tree. Larger packing containers provide more region for root increase and moisture retention. A soil mix may be appropriate, mainly for boxes or a mix of garden soil, compost, and one-of-a-type amendments. If all this sounds too

CREATING A POTTING MIX

Growing up, one in every of my desired subjects end up making the soil aggregate for our fruit wooden. I cherished playing inside the dust, however what little boy doesn't? This is wherein your children can help out and be part of this. This is the quality recipe for making homemade potting soil. You will blend identical factors of every detail depending at the soil you want. Now, permit's skip over what these factors do so that you can recognize more approximately your soil mixture and what it does.

Peat moss, moreover acknowledged sincerely as "peat," is an natural fabric that forms in waterlogged environments like peat bathrooms and swamps. It in most cases accommodates partly decomposed plant cloth, in particular sphagnum moss, and exceptional herbal don't forget amount like leaves, stems, and roots. Peat moss is significantly used in gardening, horticulture, and agriculture for its beneficial residences. Here's what peat moss does and its commonplace makes use of:

Soil Amendment: Peat moss is frequently introduced to garden soils to enhance their structure and texture. It enables to loosen compacted soils, beautify drainage in heavy soils, and boom water retention in sandy soils. Its capability to hold water and vitamins can decorate the overall fitness of vegetation.

Water Retention: One of the number one qualities of peat moss is its functionality to hold a huge amount of water. This property is useful in areas in which water is scarce or in drought-prone areas. Peat moss can assist vegetation resist dry periods at the same time as mixed with soil through manner of step by step releasing stored moisture.

Nutrient Retention: Peat moss has a excessive cation trade capacity (CEC), that would take in and release nutrients effectively. When combined with soil, it is able to assist maintain critical nutrients like nitrogen, phosphorus, and potassium,

THE LITTLE ORCHARD THAT COULD

making them to be had to plants over time.

pH Adjustment: Peat moss is slightly acidic. It can decrease the pH of alkaline soils, making them more appropriate for plants that opt for acidic situations, which includes blueberries.

Seed Starting & Propagation: Peat moss is normally used as a compo- nent in seed starting and propagation mixes. Its great texture and moisture- retaining residences create an first rate surroundings for germinating seeds and promoting the growth of extra youthful plants.

Potting Mixes: Peat moss is a critical detail in lots of business potting mixes. These mixes offer a suitable medium for potted vegetation with the resource of enhancing water retention, aeration, and nutrient availability.

Amendment for Compost: Peat moss may be incorporated into compost piles to assist stability the carbon-to-nitrogen ratio, enhance moisture retention, and beautify the overall great of the compost. It's important to be conscious that at the same time as peat moss has many benefits, its extraction and use have raised environmental problems. Harvesting peat moss can damage touchy ecosystems and release saved carbon into the ecosystem, contributing to weather trade. As an possibility, a few gardeners and specialists are exploring sustainable alternatives like coconut coir, compost, and awesome natural substances.

PERLITE

Perlite is a lightweight and porous volcanic rock normally utilized in gardening, horticulture, and hydroponics. It is created with the aid of heating volcanic glass at very immoderate temperatures, inflicting it to increase and form a white, mild-weight cloth with severa air pockets. These air wallet provide perlite unique homes, making it a precious addition to severa gardening and planting applications. Here are some of the number one makes use of and blessings of perlite:

Soil Aeration and Drainage: Perlite is frequently added to soil mixes to enhance aeration and drainage. Its porous form creates areas in the soil, considering better airflow and water movement. This allows save you soil compaction and waterlogging, that could harm the tree's roots.

Hydroponic Growing Medium: Perlite is normally used as a developing medium in hydroponic structures. Its light-weight nature allows for smooth handling and offers a suitable substrate for plant roots to anchor whilst deliberating efficient nutrient and water absorption.

Seed Starting: Perlite is carried out in seed-starting mixes to offer a mild and loose surroundings for germinating seeds. Its porosity permits prevent mildew improvement and offers younger seedlings with the critical air and water balance.

Rooting Cuttings: Gardeners often use perlite as a rooting medium for plant cuttings. Its airy texture promotes root improvement thru providing oxygen to the rooting location and preventing greater moisture buildup.

Soil Amendment: Perlite can be introduced to heavy or compacted soils to enhance their structure and drainage. Mixing perlite into the soil lets in create a more brittle and nicely-draining growing environment.

Potting Mixes: Many business potting mixes embody perlite to beautify water retention, aeration, and awesome. Perlite enables save you soil compaction in packing containers and gives a appropriate surroundings for fruit bushes to thrive.

Insulation: Perlite's insulating houses are useful for horticultural and introduction programs. It can protect tree roots from high temperature fluctuations and save you frost harm.

Roof Gardening: In rooftop gardening, perlite is sometimes utilized in developing media because of its mild-weight nature, decreasing the building shape's load.

Fireproofing: perlite is also implemented in some fireproofing programs, which encompass fireplace-resistant coatings and insulation substances.

Perlite is generally considered secure to cope with, but it's recommended to apply gloves and a mask while working with it to keep away from inhalation of high-quality debris. While perlite has many advantages, it's crucial to be aware that it has little to no nutrient-preserving potential, so it is regularly utilized in aggregate with unique soil amendments or fertilizers to offer an entire growing environment for flowers.

THE LITTLE ORCHARD THAT COULD

COMPOST

Compost is a nutrient-rich natural material created via the herbal decomposition of numerous organic materials. It's regularly called "black gold" in gardening and agriculture due to its severa advantages for soil health, tree boom, and environmental sustainability. Composting is a device that transforms herbal waste proper right into a valuable resource that may be used to beautify soil form, enhance tree growth, and reduce the quantity of waste sent to landfills. It comes from leaves and branches and then adds food scraps for numerous nutrients that timber can absorb. And remaining, we have got sand used to make the soil drain well. However, an excessive amount of sand will not preserve enough water. If you need to replace fertilizer every 12 months, you can add computer virus castings. It sounds gross, however you'll no longer eat it; your fruit wooden will. All these items you can get at your nearby garden center. So it's clean to get preserve of these form of factors. Speaking of fingers, that's what I use to mix. There's some element approximately getting your hands down in it, so pass for it. It's first rate.

FERTILIZER

Fertilizing fruit wood is vital to offer them the nutrients for healthful growth, best fruit production, and normal strength. Here are a few key elements to recognise approximately fertilizers for fruit timber:

Fruit bushes' unique nutrient requirements range based totally totally totally on their species, age, and growth degree. The number one macronutrients needed by fruit wood are nitrogen (N), phosphorus (P), and potassium

(K). However, furthermore they require secondary nutrients like calcium (Ca), magnesium (Mg), and sulfur (S), in addition to numerous micronutrients. Understanding the specific nutrient desires of your fruit tree species is important for desirable sufficient fertilization. Fruit trees advantage from balanced fertilizers that blend macronutrients and micronutrients. This enables keep away from nutrient imbalances and deficiencies. Look for fertilizers classified with an NPK ratio appropriate for fruit timber, collectively with 10-10-10 or 14-14-

14. Additionally, maintain in mind the usage of fertilizers that encompass micronutrients or encompass separate applications of micronutrient-wealthy fertilizers. The time you upload fertilizers relies upon on several factors, collectively with the tree's increase diploma, weather, and soil conditions. It isn't always uncommon to use fertilizers to

www.ingramcontent.com/pod-product-compliance
Lightning Source LLC
Chambersburg PA
CBHW062140020426
42335CB00013B/1279